# MEDICINE AND SCIENCE

NUMBER XVI OF
THE NEW YORK ACADEMY OF MEDICINE
LECTURES TO THE LAITY

# MEDICINE AND SCIENCE

## *LECTURES TO THE LAITY, NO. XVI*

THE NEW YORK ACADEMY OF MEDICINE

Iago Galdston, M. D., Editor

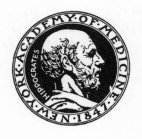

*Essay Index Reprint Series*

**BOOKS FOR LIBRARIES PRESS**
**FREEPORT, NEW YORK**

INTERNATIONAL STANDARD BOOK NUMBER:
0-8369-2122-4

LIBRARY OF CONGRESS CATALOG CARD NUMBER:
75-142679

PRINTED IN THE UNITED STATES OF AMERICA

# CONTENTS

# INTRODUCTION

The contributors to this volume, *Medicine and Science,* are men at the forefront of research; men who, in effect, are making scientific history. Their joint contribution demonstrates once again, as has been done many times in the Laity Series, that the most involved of ideas, and the most intricate information can be effectively communicated to the intelligent public without corruption of the essential facts or blatant vulgarization. In an age too prone to peddle banalities in the guise of "popularized science," these Academy lectures stand forth as distinguished and precious exceptions.

Included among the contributors to *Medicine and Science* are: Norbert Wiener, inventor of Cybernetics, Professor of Mathematics at the Massachusetts Institute of Technology, who treats of "Men, Machines and the World About," sketching in broad strokes the interrelationship between technological advances, social organization and individual well-being; all of these set in the framework of the "world about."

Hans Selye, Professor and Director of the Institute of Experimental Medicine and Surgery, at the University of Montreal, is known throughout the world for his original work on stress. He deals with "The Renaissance in Endocrinology." Building upon the pioneering works of the great French physiologist Claude Bernard and on our American pioneer, Walter B. Cannon, Professor Selye demonstrates that the living organism possesses intricate and marvelous mechanisms by which it is enabled not only to maintain "internal equilibrium" (homeostasis), but by means of which it is also capable of meeting and mastering stresses and emergencies. Beyond this, Professor Selye, reporting on his ingenious researches, shows how these mechanisms can go wrong, resulting in a variety of disorders and diseases.

David M. Levy, Professor of Clinical Psychiatry at Yale University and a pioneer in experimental psychology, deals with the intriguing problem of "The Relation of Animal Psychology to Psychiatry." This is a subject of timely interest, for it bears directly on the controversial issue of how much Pavlovianism is applicable to human psychology. Dr. Levy, in his survey, indicates how greatly the human shares in the psychological mechanisms of the lower animals, and yet he points out that it is erroneous and misleading to transpose psychological data, gathered in the setting of an animal experiment laboratory, into the realm of human psychology.

Harold G. Wolff of Cornell University Medical College presents his original research bearing on "Life Situation, Emotions and Bodily Disease." In this illuminating section, Dr. Wolff broadly extends the concepts of psychosomatic medicine, and integrates the data and experience of both psychiatric and clinical medicine.

Paul R. Burkholder, Eaton Professor of Botany, Yale University, and John E. McKeen, President of Charles Pfizer and Co., combine, in their respective and separate contributions to render a magnificent panorama of the development of antibiotic therapy. Professor Burkholder skillfully sketches the "Quest for Antibiotics," telling the story of how the academic research laboratory has been, and is, literally canvassing the four corners of the earth for new antibiotics. Mr. John E. McKeen, on the basis of his achievements as an engineer, and the administrative head of a large corporation, tells the story of the mass production of the miracle of the antibiotics. The antibiotics would have been of little profit to man or science has not modern industry succeeded in making them available in large quantities and at a cost that was fitted to every man's purse.

Interesting and instructive as these recitations are individually, they collectively yield an even more significant insight. They reflect the interdependence of modern medicine on the totality of science. Hence the warrant for the title.

This book must prove of interest to the laity, physicians, biologists, the public health worker, the social worker, the nursing specialist, the specialized scientist and indeed to every person who seeks to *understand, as well as to know,* what is taking place in medicine today.

HOWARD R. CRAIG, M.D.

# MEDICINE AND SCIENCE

# MEN, MACHINES, AND
# THE WORLD ABOUT

## By Norbert Wiener, Ph. D.

I WANT to point historically to the various things that got me interested in the problems of man, machines, and the world about, because they are relevant to the various things I shall have to say about the present status of the problem.

There were two converging streams of ideas that brought me into cybernetics. One of them was the fact that in the last war, or when it was manifestly coming, at any rate before Pearl Harbor, when we were not yet in the conflict, I tried to see if I could find some niche in the war effort.

In that particular problem, I looked for something to do, and found it in connection with automatic computing machines. Automatic computing machines, of what is called an analogy sort, in which physical quantities are measured and not numbers counted, had already been made very successfully by Professor Vannevar Bush, but there were certain gaps in the theory.

One of the gaps I can express mathematically by saying that these machines could do ordinary differential equations but not partial differential equations. I shall express it physically by the fact that these machines could work in one dimension, namely, time, but not in any efficient way in two dimensions, or three.

Now, it occurred to me that (a) the use of television had shown us a way to represent two or more dimensions on one device; and (b) that the previous device which measured quantities should be replaced by a more precise sort of device that counted numbers.

These were not only my own ideas, but at any rate, they were ideas that I had then, and I communicated them in a memorandum to Vannevar Bush, who was in charge of scientific war planning for the entire country. The report that I gave was, in many ways, not in all, a substantial account of the present situation with automatic computing machines. Thus, I had already become familiar with the idea of the machine which does its arithmethic by making choices on the basis of previous choices, and these on the basis of previous choices, and so on, according to a schedule furnished to the machine by punched tape, or by magnetized tape, or other methods of the sort.

The other thing which led me to this work was the problem that I actually got put into in war work. It turned out that at that time Professor Bush did not feel that this contribution was immediate enough to have been effective in the last war. So I looked around for another thing, and the great question that was being discussed at that time was antiaircraft defense. It was at the time of the Battle of England and the existence of the United States as a combatant country—the survival of anybody to combat Germany—seemed to depend on antiaircraft defense.

The antiaircraft gun is a very interesting type of instrument. In the First World War, the antiaircraft gun had been developed as a firing instrument, but one still used range tables directly by hand for firing the gun. That meant, essentially, that one had to do all the computation while the plane was flying overhead, and, naturally, by the time you got in position to do something about it, the plane had already done something about it, and was not there.

It became evident—and this was long before the work that I did—by the end of the First World War, and certainly by the period between the two, that the essence of the problem was to do all the computation in advance and embody it in instruments which could pick up the observations of the plane and fuse them in the proper way to get the necessary result to aim the gun and to aim it, not at the plane, but sufficiently ahead of the plane, so that the shell and the plane would arrive at the same time as induction. That led to some very interesting mathematical theories.

I had some ideas that turned out to be useful there, and I was put to work with a friend of mine, Julian Bigelow. Very soon we ran into the following problem: the anti-aircraft gun is not an isolated instrument. While it can be fired by radar, the equivalent and obvious method of firing it is to have a gun pointer. The gun pointer is a human element; this human element is joined with the mechanical elements. The actual fire control is a system involving human beings and machines at the same time. It must be reduced, from an engineering point of view, to a single structure, which means either a human interpretation of the machine, or a mechanical interpretation of the operator, or both. We were forced—both for the man firing the gun and for the aviator himself—to replace them in our studies by appropriate machines. The question arose: How would we make a machine to simulate a gun pointer, and what troubles would one expect with the situation?

There is a certain sort of control apparatus used for controlling speed in the governors of steam engines, that is used for controlling direction in the ship-steering apparatus, which is called a negative feedback apparatus. In the ship-steering apparatus, the quartermaster who turns the wheel does not move the rudder directly. The rudder is much too heavy in the modern ship for a dozen quartermasters to do that. What he does is to move an element in the steering-engine house which is connected with the tiller of the ship by another element. The difference between the two positions is then conveyed to the steering engines of the two sides of the ship to regulate the admission of steam in the port or starboard steering engine. The steering engine moves the rudder head, the tiller, in such a way as to cancel this interval that has been placed between this moving element and the rudder head, and in doing that it recloses the valves and moves the rudder with the ship. In other words, the rudder is moved by something representing the difference between the commanded position and in its own actual position. That is called negative feedback.

This negative feedback, however, has its diseases. There is a definite pathology to it which was already discussed —you will be rather astonished at the date—in 1868, by the great physicist, Clerk Maxwell, in a paper in the Proceedings of the Royal Society in London. If the feedback of the rudder, or the governor, is too intense, the apparatus will shoot past the neutral position a little further than it was originally past it on one side—will shoot further past it on the other—and will go into oscillation.

Since we thought that the simplest way that we could

explain human control was by a feedback, we wondered whether this disease would occur. We went with the following question to our friend, Dr. Arturo Rosenblueth, a physiologist, who was then Cannon's right-hand man in the Harvard Medical School: Is there any nervous disease known in which a person trying to accomplish a task starts swinging wider and wider, and is unable to finish it? For example, I reach for my cigar. I suppose the ordinary way I control my action is so as to reduce the amount by which the cigar has not yet been picked up. Is that disease of excessive oscillation known?

The answer was most definitely that this disease is known. It has exactly the symptoms named. It occurs in the pathology of the cerebellum, the little brain. It is known as purpose tremor or cerebellar tremor.

Well, that gave us the lead. It looked as if a common pattern could be given to account for human behavior and controlled machine behavior in this case, and that it depended on negative feedback.

That was one of the leads we had. The other lead went back to the study of the automatic controlling machine, the automatic computing machine.

In the first place, automatic computing machinery is of no value except for one thing: its speed. It is more expensive than the ordinary desk machine, enormously more. You do not get anything out of it unless you use it at high speed. But to use a machine at high speed, it is necessary to see that every operation it carries out is carried out at a corresponding speed. If you mix in slow stages with fast stages of the machine, the slow stages always win out. They more nearly govern the behavior of the machine than the fast stages. Therefore, the commands given to a high-speed computing machine cannot be given by hand, while the machine is running. They must be built in in advance to what is called a taping, like punched cards, like punched tape, like magnetic tape, or something of the sort; and your machine must not only control the numbers and their combinations, but the scheduling of operations. Your machine must be a logical machine.

There again we found a great similarity to what a human being was doing. The human nervous system, it is perfectly true, does not exhaust all of human control activity. There is, without any doubt, a control activity in man that goes through hormones, that goes through the blood, and so on. But, as far as the nervous system works, the individual fibers come very near to showing an "all or none" action, that is, they fire or they do not fire; they do not fire halfway. If your individual fibers leading to a given fiber and connected to it by what is known as a synapse, fire in the proper combination—perhaps at least as many as a certain number—and if certain so-called inhibitory fibers do not interrupt them, the outgoing fibers fire. Otherwise they do not.

This is an operation of connected switching extremely like the connected switching of the automatic computing machine. This led us to another comparison between the nervous system and the computing machine, and led us, furthermore, to the idea that since the nervous system is not only a computing machine but a control machine, that we may make very general control machines, working on the successive switching basis and much more like the control machine part, the scheduling part of a computing machine, than we might otherwise have thought possible.

In particular, it seemed to us a very hopeful thing to make an automatic feedback control apparatus in which the feedback itself was carried out, in large measure, by successive switching operations such as one finds either in the nervous system or in the computing machine.

It was the fusion of these two ideas, each of which has a human or animal side and has a machine side, which led to *Cybernetics*. That book I wrote in response to a request from a French publisher, and I chose the name, for I felt that this particular combination of ideas could not be left too long unbaptized, took it from the Greek word Κυβερνᾶν meaning to govern, as essentially the art of the steersman.

From here on, I can go ahead in very many ways. The first thing that I want to say is that the feedback mechanisms are not only well known to occur in the voluntary actions of the human body, but that they are necessary for its very life.

A few years ago, Professor Henderson of Harvard wrote a book entitled *The Fitness of the Environment*. Anybody who has read that book must regard it as very much of a miracle that any organism can live, and particularly a human organism. Man cannot exist over any variety of temperatures. For that matter, there is no active life, certainly not above the boiling point and below the freezing point, and most planets probably do not have temperatures lying in that convenient range. When I say "boiling point" and "freezing point," I mean of water, because water is a very distinct and special sort of chemical substance.

Now, even a fish cannot exist at the boiling point. It can exist at something like our own temperature to something around the freezing point, perhaps a little bit below, but not much below.

We cannot do anything like that. We either have a chill or a fever if we get near it. The temperature at which life is possible does not vary for man for any extended period of time. It certainly does not vary much over ten degrees, and practically varies much less than that. Again, we must live under constant conditions of saltiness of our blood, of urea concentration in our blood, and so on.

How do we do this? The idea goes back to Claude Bernard and was developed very much by Cannon. We are full of what is called homeostatic mechanisms, which are mechanisms like thermostats. A homeostat is a mechanism which keeps certain bodily conditions within a narrow range. One of those homeostats, located partly, at least, in the medulla, regulates temperature. Another one regulates breathing. Another one of them regulates urea concentration. That is the apparatus of the kidneys. There are not only a few, but many, many such controls.

Now, such control is like the house thermostat. The house thermostat, if you remember it, is a piece of apparatus which has a little thermometer in it made of two pieces of metal. It makes a contact at one temperature and breaks it at others, and it regulates the admission of oil to the furnace and the ignition of that oil. The interesting thing is it has its own pathology. Many of you people must know that.

We have a house in which there is a thermostat which some brilliant architect placed in the only room in the house with a fireplace. The result is that if we want to cool the house in winter, we light the fire because we give false information to the thermostat that the house is warm and the thermostat turns out the furnace fire.

I might point out that a similar behavior in the human thermostat might cause chills or might cause fever. I am going to depart a little from the main part of the formal talk, because this thing is medically very interesting.

There are certain diseases—I am not going into a characterization of these, because I am not going to commit myself before so many doctors—in which the production of certain substances, say cells, the density of certain cells in the blood, as in leukemia, is increasing steadily. However, this steady increase is rather a regular thing in the disease. The actual rate of production and destruction of the cells is much, much higher than the rate of increase. That might be due, conceivably, to an independent disease of production or of destruction, but I do not think so, because if these two phenomena give you big quantities that are nearly the same, a relatively small change in one will throw this difference out badly and produce a great irregularity in their difference. That is what would have happened if we had no homeostat. I do not think that is what happens. I think that the regularity of the procedure is an indication that we have a homeostat which is working, but working at the wrong level, as if the spring of the house thermostat were changing. That is an idea which is entirely tentative, but which may have serious consequences for medicine.

There is another side to this which is also interesting. The homeostats in the body that I have spoken of are built into the human body. Can we make a homeostat that is partly in the body and partly outside? The answer is definitely yes.

Dr. Bickford at the Mayo Clinic—and he has been followed in this by Dr. Verzeano in the Cushing Veterans Hospital in Framingham—has made an apparatus which takes the brain waves of the electroencephalogram and divides them up, using the total amount that has passed for a stated time, to inject anesthetic either into the vein or into a mask. The procedure is this: as the patient goes under, the brain waves become less active; the injections become less, as less injection is actually needed to keep the level of unconsciousness. In this way, anesthesia can be kept at a reasonably constant level for hours. Here you have a homeostat which is a manufactured one. I do not believe that this is the last example in medicine. I think that the administration of drugs by homeostats which are monitored by their physiologic consequences is a field which has a great future. However, I say this tentatively.

Now, so far I have been talking about man. Let us go to the machine. Where will we find a case where a homeostatic machine is particularly desirable?

Chemistry is an interesting case in point. A chemical factory is generally full of pipes carrying acids, or alkalis, or explosives—at any rate, substances dangerous to work with. When certain thermometers reach certain readings, and certain pressures have been reached, and so on, somebody turns certain valves. He had better turn the right valves, particularly in something like an oil-cracking plant or atomic energy plant, where we are dealing with radio-active materials.

If he has to turn valves on the basis of readings, then, as in the antiaircraft gun, we can build in in advance the combinations which should turn valves as distinguished from those which should not. The valves may be turned through amplifiers, through what is essentially computing apparatus, by the reading of the instruments themselves, the instruments or sense organs.

You may say, "Very good, but you have to have a man to provide for emergencies."

By the way, it is extremely desirable not to have people in a factory that is likely to explode. People are expensive to replace, and besides we have certain elementary humanitarian instincts.

22

The question is: Is a man likely to use better emergency judgment than a machine? The answer is no. The reason for that is this: any emergency you can think of, you can provide for in your computing and control apparatus. If before the time of the emergency, you cannot think of what to do, during the emergency you are almost certain to make a wrong decision. If you cannot figure out a reasonable course of conduct in advance, you simply do not find that the Lord will give you the right thing to do when the emergency comes. Emergencies are provided for in times of peace. I also mean by that, emergencies like the falling of an atomic bomb, about which I may or may not have something to say later.

Then, for perfectly legitimate or even humanitarian reasons, the automatic control system is coming in in chemical industry and in other especially dangerous industries. However, the same technics that make possible the automatic assembly line for automobiles, perhaps one automatic assembly line in the textiles industry, and possibly even in dozens of other industries.

The interesting thing is this: that while the successive orders that you give can be almost indefinitely varied in a machine, the instruments which elaborate successive orders are practically standard, no matter what you are doing. These are two variables: one is the quasihuman hands to which the central machine leads, and the other is the sequence of orders put in.

To change from one set of orders, say, from one make of car to another, or to change from one style of body to another, in an assembly line, it is not necessary to alter the order-giving machine. It is enough to alter the particular taping of that machine.

I suppose a good many of you have seen the movie,

"Cheaper by the Dozen." In that movie, what I consider to be the leading idea of the Gilbraiths is completely missed, as it would be in most movies. The Gilbraiths had the idea that man was not working at anything like his full efficiency in his ordinary operations. They thought that families of a dozen were not had by people simply because of human stupidity in the performance of daily tasks, and that this could be avoided by a better ordering of those tasks. That was the motive behind the large family. That was the motive behind the systematic bringing up of those children.

However, when you have simplified a task by reducing it to a routine of consecutive procedures, you have done the same sort of thing that you need to do to put the task on a tape and run the procedure by a completely automatic machine. The problem of industrial management and the systematic handling of ordinary detail by the Gilbraiths, and so forth, is almost the same problem as the taping of a control machine; so that instead of actually improving the conditions of the worker, their advance has tended to telescope the worker out of the picture. That is a very important thing, because it is a procedure taking place now.

I want to say that we are facing a new industrial revolution. The first industrial revolution represented the replacement of the energy of man and of animals by the energy of the machine. The steam engine was its symbol. That has gone so far that there is nothing that steam and the bulldozer cannot do. There is no rate at which pure pick-and-shovel work can be paid in this country which will guarantee a man's doing it willingly. It is simply economically impossible to compete with a bulldozer for bulldozer work.

The new industrial revolution which is taking place now consists primarily in replacing human judgment and discrimination at low levels by the discrimination of the machine. The machine appears now, not as a source of power, but as a source of control and a source of communication. We communicate with the machine and the machine communicates with us. Machines communicate with one another. Energy and power are not the proper concepts to describe this new phenomenon.

If we, in a small way, make human tasks easier by replacing them with a machine execution of the task, and in a large way eliminate the human element in these tasks, we may find we have essentially burned incense before the machine god. There is a very real danger in this country in bowing down before the brass calf, the idol, which is the gadget. I know a great engineer who never thinks further than the construction of the gadget and never thinks of the question of the integration between the gadget and human beings in society. If we allow things to have a reasonably slow development, then the introduction of the gadget as it naturally comes, may hurt us enough to provoke a salutary response. So, we realize we cannot worship the gadget and sacrifice the human being to it, but a situation is easily possible in which we may incur a disaster.

Let us suppose that we get into a full-scale war with Russia. I think that Korea, if nothing else, has shown us that modern war means nothing without the infantry. The trouble of occupying Korea is serious enough. The problem of occupying China and Russia staggers the imagination.

We shall have to prepare to do this, if we go to war, at the same time as we have to keep up an industrial production to feed the Army. I mean feed it with munitions as well as with ordinary food and ordinary equipment, a job second to none in history. We shall have to do a maximum production job with a labor market simply scraped to the bottom, and that means the automatic machine.

A war of that sort would mean that we would be putting a large part of our best engineering talent in developing the machine, within two months, probably. It happens that the people who do this sort of job are there. They are the people who were trained in electronic work in the last war when they worked with radar. We are further on with the automatic machine than we were with radar at Pearl Harbor.

Therefore, the situation is that probably two to three years will see the automatic factory well understood and its use beginning to accelerate production. Five years from now will see in the automatic assembly line something of which we possess the complete know-how, and of which we possess a vast backlog of parts.

Furthermore, social reforms do not get made in war. At the end of such a war, we shall find ourselves with a tremendous backlog of parts and know-how, which is extremely tempting to anybody who wants to make a quickie fortune and get out from under, and leave the rest of the community to pick up the pieces. That may very well happen. If that does happen, heaven help us, because we will have an unemployment compared with which the great depression was a nice little joke.

Well, you see the picture drawing together. I suppose one of the things that you people would like would be consolation. Gentlemen, there is no Santa Claus! If we want to live with the machine, we must understand the machine, we must not worship the machine. We must make a great many changes in the way we live with other people. We must value leisure. We must turn the great leaders of business, of industry, of politics, into a state of mind in which they will consider the leisure of people as their business and not as something to be passed off as none of their business.

We shall have to do this unhampered by slogans which fitted a previous stage in society but which do not fit the present.

We shall have to do this unhampered by the creeping paralysis of secrecy which is engulfing our government, because secrecy simply means that we are unable to face situations as they really exist. The people who have to control situations are as yet in no position to handle them.

We shall have to realize that while we may make the machines our gods and sacrifice men to machines, we do not have to do so. If we do so, we deserve the punishment of idolators. It is going to be a difficult time. If we can live through it and keep our heads, and if we are not annihilated by war itself and our other problems, there is a great chance of turning the machine to human advantage, but the machine itself has no particular favor for humanity.

It is possible to make two kinds of machines (I shall not go into the details): the machine whose taping is determined once and for all, and the machine whose taping is continually being modified by experience. The second machine can, in some sense, learn.

Gentlemen, the moral problem of the machine differs in no way from the old moral problem of magic. The fact that the machine follows the law of Nature and that magic is supposed to be outside of Nature is not an interesting distinction. Sorcery was condemned in the Middle Ages. In those ages certain modern types of gadgeteer would have been hanged or burned as a sorcerer. An interesting thing is that the Middle Ages to a certain extent—oh, I don't mean in its love for the flame, but in its condemnation of the gadgeteer—would have been right; namely, sorcery was not the use of the supernatural, but the use of human power for other purposes than the greater glory of God.

Now, I am not theistic when I say the greater glory of God. I mean by God some end to which we can give a justifiable human value. I say that the medieval attitude is the attitude of the fairy tale in many things, but the attitude of the fairy tale is very wise in many things that are relevant to modern life.

If you have the machine which grants you your wish, then you must pay attention to the old fairy tale of the three wishes, which tells you that if you do make a wish which is likely to be granted, you had better be very sure that it is what you want and not what you think you want.

You know Jacob's story of the monkey's paw, the talisman. An old couple came into possession of this, and learned that it would grant them three wishes. The first wish was for two hundred pounds. Immediately, a man appeared from the factory to say that their boy had been crushed in the machinery, and although the factory recognized no responsibility, they were ready to give a solatium of two hundred pounds.

After this they wished the boy back again, and his ghost appeared.

Then they wished the ghost to go away, and there they were left with nothing but a dead son. That is the story.

This is a piece of folklore; but the problem is quite as relevant to the machine as to any piece of magic.

However, a machine can learn. Here the folklore parallel is to the tale of the fisherman and the genie. You all know the story. The fisherman opens a bottle which he has

*Men, Machines, and the World About*

found on the shore, and the genie appears. The genie threatens him with vengeance for his own imprisonment. The fisherman talks the genie back into the bottle. Gentlemen, when we get into trouble with the machine, we cannot talk the machine back into the bottle.

*29*

# THE RENAISSANCE
# IN ENDOCRINOLOGY*

*By Hans Selye, M. D., Ph. D., D. Sc., F. R. S. (C.)
and Paul Rosch, M. D.*

WHEN I was chosen by this Academy to speak to you about the "renaissance in endocrinology," I must admit that I was both honored and dismayed. No doubt it was flattering to learn that your program committee should think of me in this connection, but I seriously doubt that I shall be able to do justice to this imposing title.

Yet the term renaissance or "rebirth" does appear to be eminently applicable to the recent advances which characterize contemporary endocrinology and, indeed, medicine as a whole. Within the comparatively short period of fifty years, the physician's arsenal against disease has been almost completely renovated. In the first decade of this century, a list of ten drugs, thought to be the most important and useful, prominently featured mercury, iron, iodine, and alcohol (Castiglioni, 1947). Since then, and especially in the past ten years, the advent of hormones, antibiotics, radioactive compounds, etc., has necessitated a new ap-

* This address was presented by H. Selye, on the basis of lecture notes from which P. Rosch prepared the text reproduced here in print.

proach to the art of Hippocrates, and has stimulated widespread interest in the study of the nature and cause of disease in general.

It seems to me that advances in medicine may be considered as being of two main types—technical, and philosophic. The technical advances include the application of newer scientific methods and tools to the problems of research. They are responsible for such advances as improved surgical techniques, increasing yields in the extraction or synthesis of drugs, and for many of the useful newer devices such as the mechanical respirator used in poliomyelitis or the artificial kidney employed in the treatment of uremia. This type of progress may be viewed as the result of a *search for knowledge.*

On the other hand, are advances rooted in the sincere desire for a better understanding of nature and a fundamental evaluation of our discoveries. Such philosophic advances are aspects of the *search for wisdom.*

In the long run, the latter is more practical, for, as Tennyson said,

"Knowledge comes, but wisdom lingers."

Or, as Cowper has distinguished,

"Knowledge and wisdom, far from being one,
Have oft-time no connexion. Knowledge dwells
In heads replete with thoughts of other men;
Wisdom in minds attentive to their own.
Knowledge, a rude unprofitable mass,
The mere materials with which wisdom builds,
Till smooth'd and squar'd and fitted to its place,
Does but encumber whom it seems t'enrich.
Knowledge is proud that he has learned so much;
Wisdom is humble that he knows no more."

Actually, both the search for knowledge and the search for wisdom are but two aspects of the study of life, and there are many ways of approaching this study.

There is the tabulation of simple facts, such as the registration of structural detail or of biochemical changes produced by an experimental intervention. This work is safe; it is the *book-keeping of Nature.*

There is the descriptive characterization of complex facts, such as clinical syndromes, or intricate tissue reactions. This work is inspired; it is the *landscaping of Nature.*

Finally, there is the correlation of facts into a unified system, a Science. For the explorer of Nature this yields a practically useful (though not necessarily complete or even correct) map of navigation. It helps him to remember the points he has seen and to discover new ones along the roads of abstractions which connect them. This work is creative; it may lead far astray, but apart from procreation, this is the closest man can come to the *making of Nature.*

It is in this last approach to the study of life that our own modest efforts have been directed, and perhaps we may take this opportunity to review briefly our attempt at a correlation of what seemed to be widely diversified observations, and to explain how this concept relates to some of the newer advances.

The "renaissance in endocrinology" may be thought of as being heralded by the new "era of ACTH and cortisone." It is somewhat embarrassing to have been asked to speak to you on this subject, inasmuch as I did not discover these substances, nor was I the first to use them. My only connection with this field was the formulation of the concept of the "adaptation syndrome," in which ACTH and cortisone and other "corticoids" play a vital role. This syndrome is a natural but complex defense reaction of the body, and helps to protect us against many diseases.

Our further investigations into the study of this natural reactive pattern of body defenses led to the discovery that certain disorders can be brought about when there is an insufficiency, imbalance, or similar derangement of ACTH or corticoid actions during the "adaptation syndrome." Accordingly, we called these "diseases of adaptation."

Among these illnesses produced by failure to adapt correctly are the rheumatic diseases, of which some forms of arthritis are excellent examples. Inasmuch as the adrenal cortex governs corticoid production, and derangements in this process can produce "diseases of adaptation," such as arthritis, it seemed logical to us that this endocrine gland should have an important part in determining whether such conditions will or will not develop, under given circumstances.

Experimental studies designed to test the validity of this assumption proved rewarding; through them, a clearer insight into the true nature of these disorders began to evolve early in the 1940's. They also helped to substantiate many heretofore vague hypotheses, and paved the way for the application, to the problems of clinical medicine, of the stress concept in general, and of the "adaptive hormones" in particular.

### THE GENERAL ADAPTATION SYNDROME

With this background in mind, it might be profitable for us now to review, very briefly, some of the principal tenets of this "general adaptation syndrome," in order to facilitate an understanding of its relationship to the concept of disorders of adaptation, and especially the rheumatic allergic diseases.

## Hans Selye and Paul Rosch

A series of animal experiments, performed in the course of 1935-1936, showed us that the organism responds in a stereotyped manner to a variety of widely different agents such as infections, intoxications, trauma, nervous strain, temperature extremes, muscular fatigue or X-irradiation. Each of these agents, to be sure, had its own specific effects, in many cases, diametrically opposed (e.g., heat causes dilatation of small blood vessels, while cold brings about vasoconstriction), but common to all was the fact that they placed the body in a state of stress, and that the organism responded in the same stereotyped manner to this stress, regardless of the nature of the agent provoking it. Thus, the resultant effect was the summation and superimposition of the specific actions of the "stressor" upon the general reactive pattern elicited by what I called "nonspecific stress."

Hence, exposure to noxious stimuli induces a state of stress, and the nonspecific adaptive reaction which characterizes the body's response is in the nature of a "call to arms" of the organism's defenses. It was named the "alarm reaction." Further results indicated that this was merely the first development of a much more prolonged "general adaptation syndrome," which comprises three phases: the "alarm reaction," in which adaptation has not yet been acquired; the "stage of resistance," in which adaptation is optimal; and finally, the "stage of exhaustion," in which the acquired adaptation is lost again.

Adaptability is probably the most distinctive characteristic of life. In maintaining the independence and individuality of natural units, none of the great forces of inanimate matter are as successful as that alertness and adaptability to change which we designate as life—and the loss of which is death. Indeed there is perhaps even a certain parallelism between the degree of aliveness and the extent of adaptability in every animal—in every man [Selye, 1950].

It should be emphasized that I said "degree of aliveness" and "extent of adaptability," since inanimate systems can also adapt to certain changes in their surroundings, but even the most perfect man-made automaton cannot approximate the adaptability of the simplest living organism. It seems to me that it is precisely that extraordinary quality of certain aggregates of matter, which endows all parts of their structure with the power of self-maintenance in the face of so many qualitatively different aggressors, that we empirically came to consider Life. What machine could assess whether it should attack or run away from its enemy, could forage for its fuel, develop an ethical order permitting it to exist in a co-operative society with its congeners in order to fight common dangers, or heal a scratch on its surface. No doubt complex mechanical devices have been made to imitate some of these properties of Life and these could be further perfected, but my imagination bogs at the thought that even the adaptability of the simplest ameba could ever be reproduced by man using inanimate ingredients.

Thus everything in life, even its seemingly fundamental dissimilarity from the Inanimate, is a matter of degree—that is why no other generalization about life can be wholly true [Selye, 1951].

Yet, as I said in the introduction, the progress of medical research is largely dependent upon theories and generalizations, even if they are correct only to a certain degree. Let us, therefore, proceed now with our attempt to develop a unified theory of disease in general, on the basis of what we called the "stress concept."

The manner by which stress initiates the biologic "chain reaction" of adaptation is unknown, but a dual course may be assumed. One response leads to *damage* or "shock," possibly through nervous stimuli, deficiencies, or toxic metabolites. The other, its inseparable companion, is concerned with *defense;* it depends largely upon the activities of the pituitary and adrenal glands. We will deal mainly with the latter, since we believe that much information of practical value for the sick can be learned by emulating (if possible with improvements) the body's own techniques of defense.

In conditions of stress, the pituitary is stimulated to secrete what are known as corticotrophic hormones. These influence the adrenal to produce two main types of adrenocortical hormones or "corticoids."

The somatotrophic or "growth" hormone of the pituitary (STH) acts mainly by sensitizing tissues to "mineralo-corticoids" such as desoxycorticosterone. The adrenocorticotrophic hormone (ACTH) causes primarily a secretion of "gluco-corticoids," of which cortisone is one example. These two types of hormones are secreted by the adrenal cortex in large amounts under stress.

The mineralo-corticoids (desoxycorticosterone-like) and the gluco-corticoids (cortisone-like) have many opposing effects. The former may be viewed as preparing the body for fight, the latter, for surrender. The mineralo-corticoids act so as to put up a barricade of connective tissue against the stressor agent, the gluco-corticoids, to continue the analogy, remove all obstacles from his path. Deficiencies or imbalances in corticoid output caused by stress lead to "diseases of adaptation," which, as you can see now, are really due to maladaptation. In a sense, one might say that they are the results of errors in assessing the relative expediency of defense, or tactical withdrawal, before the foe.

Soon after we observed that arthritic and other rheumatic disorders could be produced by DCA overdosage in animals, it was noted that these same diseases could be treated by DCA-inhibiting corticoids, of which cortisone is the best known example. Interestingly, this latter observation, undoubtedly the most important one along these lines up to date, was made by another group (Hench et al., 1949), working along entirely separate lines. Yet, the results significantly strengthened and supported the legitimacy of this type of thinking and demonstrated its applicability to clinical problems.

To sum up, as you can see in the figure presented below, a stressor agent acts directly (thick black line) and indirectly on the body. The direct effects of each stressor are different, but the general nonspecific reaction induced by stressors is always the same and influences the body via the production of STH, which causes mineralo-corticoid secretion, and ACTH, which is responsible for the stimulation of antagonistically acting gluco-corticoids (shown by cross hatched lines). Derangements in production of either of these four substances result in "diseases of adaptation" as we have explained above.

This concept, which aims at a unification of ideas, is an attempt at something rather new in the study of disease. Heretofore, we used to think and plan along two main lines. One dealt with causal therapy and suggested the use of antibiotics, surgery, etc., either to kill the pathogen or to cut it out. The other therapeutic approach to sickness was symptomatic, such as utilization of aspirin to deaden the pain of a headache regardless of its cause. These are both practical, useful, methods of combating illness. We have

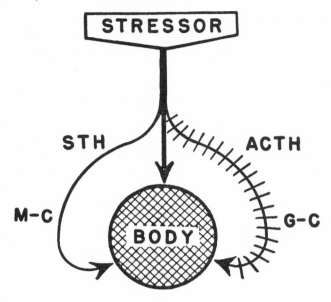

FIGURE 1

Fɪɢ. 1.—*Schematic drawing illustrating principal mechanisms effective during exposure to stress.* Body = the whole organism, or any part of it, which is directly affected by a stressor agent; STH = somato-trophic hormone; ACTH = adrenocorticotrophic hormone; M-C = mineralo-corticoid hormones; G-C = gluco-corticoid hormones; simple arrow = stimu-lates; cross-hatched arrow = inhibits. For explana-tion see text. (Slightly modified after Selye, *Annual Report on Stress—1951.* Acta Inc. Medical Publishers, Montreal.)

added the general adaptive theory in the hope of integrat-ing and correlating previous work and offering a new ap-proach to the treatment and understanding of disease, through the search for a "stress factor" or "mal-adaptation factor," which would be common to many seemingly different types of disorders. We hope by this to gain insight into the nature of certain illnesses and perhaps develop a cure or prophylaxis for them.

There is need for some unified concept in medicine today. We have had almost no great theorists in this field for many years now; at least none that could be compared to the great creators of new schools of thought, who worked in Europe during the nineteenth and the first part of the twentieth century, such as:

Pasteur           (1822-1895)—who founded bacteriology and serology

Claude Bernard (1813-1878)—responsible for the development of experimental medicine and the concept of the "milieu intérieur," which was developed in our time by Cannon as the theory of "homeostasis"

Virchow          (1821-1902)—who inspired the study of pathological anatomy and histology

Ehrlich          (1854-1915)—the pioneer in chemotherapy

Pavlov           (1849-1936)—who developed the importance of the conditioned reflex and the relationship between mind and body

Freud            (1856-1939)—who brought to fruition the importance of psychosomatic medicine and psychoanalysis.

However, this golden era of thinkers soon began to degenerate, perhaps because scientists were dazed by the extraordinary efficiency of theories as guides to knowledge. It was forgotten that in the natural sciences, the mere contemplation of potential new pathways into the unknown is of little value in itself. It must be followed by the painstaking experimental exploration of their viability. Disregard of this fundamental truth eventually left Europe with a great excess of "armchair philosophers" given to vague speculation, pompous dialectic theorizing and, eventually, futile priority squabbles.

It is, unfortunately, just at this time that large numbers of young American students and scientists began to visit Europe, attracted by the glorious past of its great universities. Too many of them fell into the hands of masters who attempted in vain to give a semblance of authority to their dialectic teachings, by exaggerating the importance of their rank through academic pomp and circumstance. These young men returned to the United States with a definite aversion to any aspect of science except the search for facts whose value was immediately assessable.

Thus the pendulum began to swing toward the other extreme, the abhorrence of theory. "Pure objectivity" became the fashionable slogan in medical research and this was coupled with an unreasonable fear that any thought expressed in print might subsequently be proven to be wrong. Even today many a scientist concludes an extensive paper, replete with tables and statistical calculations, by stating—often with an air of self-righteousness—that: "the facts reported are certainly correct, but no attempt is made to draw any conclusions from them." This is undoubtedly very honest and no one can question the moral virtue of such investigators, but one may doubt their wisdom. What is the purpose of establishing something with the greatest degree of probability if one ignores its significance? Are not many of those who consistently reject the expression of opinions in science too much concerned with the importance of their own personal prestige? Is it worthwhile

to sacrifice the pleasure of trying really to understand
Nature for the superficial glory of creating a semblance of
personal infallibility?

Undoubtedly, purely objective and descriptive research
and the dispassionate registration of facts may lead to the
acquisition of important knowledge. Indeed—with adequate financial support—even the mere screening of all
possibilities can force Nature to reveal some of her secrets.
I must admit (although this is very distasteful to me) that
many technical advances have been made in this fashion.
However, those who use this kind of approach do not try
to conquer Nature by love and understanding, but merely
wish to rape her by force. They may possess her substance,
but not her spirit.

Our modest attempt to explore the "adaptation syndrome" has not brought forth very much, as yet, that is
immediately applicable to the treatment of sickness, but
we like to think that it has contributed its share to the
"rebirth" of medicine, through its attempt to stimulate
thought and again demonstrate the value of approaching
research problems with a definite theoretic formulation.

#### THE VALUE OF A THEORY

It is well to realize that "our facts must be correct; our
theories need not be if they help us to discover important
new facts" (Selye, 1950). Indeed, once a theory says "nothing but the truth and all the truth" about a certain subject,
it has lost its heuristic value and then it is no longer a
theory, but merely the enunciation of a fact.

The best theory is that which necessitates the minimum
amount of assumptions to unite the maximum number of
facts, since it is most likely to possess the power of assimi-

lating new facts from the unknown without damage to its own structure.

It is perhaps insufficiently realized by many that even a faulty theory may be of great value. Pierre Marie's concept of the relationship between the pituitary and acromegaly was directly opposite to what we now know to be true. He found that acromegalic giants had pituitary tumors and concluded that they became tall because their pituitary was destroyed by disease. Actually we now know that such tumorous glands produce a great excess of somatotrophic or "growth" hormone and that this is responsible for the disproportionate increase in the growth of these patients. Surely, no theory could have united the facts observed by Pierre Marie more incorrectly than that which he enunciated. Nevertheless, the very fact that he called attention to some relationship between gigantism and the pituitary was of immense value and stimulated much research, eventually culminating in the discovery of the somatotrophic or "growth" hormone.

The key that opens the door usually also serves to lock it, the most important thing is to find the key that fits the lock of the door we wish to use.

We tried to outline the concept of the "general adaptation syndrome" and the manner in which derangements in the adaptive mechanism to stress may cause disease. As it stands, our map of these uncharted parts of medicine is certainly both incorrect and incomplete, but let us hope that it possesses that critical degree of truthfulness which stimulates to rectify the misdrawn boundary lines and to fill out the spaces where hitherto unexplored territories are shown to lie. This hope is our only justification and apology for having accepted the great honor of participating in this lecture series.

# The Renaissance in Endocrinology

REFERENCES

Castiglioni, Arturo (1947), *A History of Medicine.* New York: Alfred A. Knopf, p. 1055.

Cowper, William (1934), The Task. *Cowper's Poetical Works,* Book VI, lines 88-99. London: Oxford University Press.

Hench, P. S., Kendall, E. C., Slocumb, C. H. and Polley, H. F. (1949), *Proceedings of the Staff Meeting of the Mayo Clinic,* 24:181.

Selye, Hans (1950), *Stress.* Montreal: Acta Inc. Medical Publishers.

—— (1951), *Annual Report on Stress.* Montreal: Acta Inc. Medical Publishers.

Tennyson, Alfred (1898), Locksley Hall. *The Poetic and Dramatic Works of Alfred Lord Tennyson.* Cambridge Edition. Cambridge: The Riverside Press, line 141.

# THE RELATION OF ANIMAL PSYCHOLOGY TO PSYCHIATRY

## By David M. Levy, M.D.

### OUR ATTITUDE TOWARDS ANIMAL PSYCHOLOGY

ALTHOUGH we see certain resemblances of animal behavior and our own, we regard our own behavior as infinitely more complicated and superior, befitting the higher order of man in the animal scale. The complexity of our order, judged by any one of the products of civilization, seems to set us so far apart from the animal world that, however "human" many animal anecdotes appear to be, most of us may wonder or be amused, but never interested to the point of seriously incorporating such stories into the process of theorizing about human psychology. The same holds true for animal studies that have scientific validity. Though we cannot assign them to the category of harmless anecdotes full of the flaws of human projections, like stories of infants by proud parents, they have never become an integral part of our clinical thinking.

Our way of disregarding studies of animal psychology, or at least of keeping them in a separate compartment when we formulate theories in psychiatry, does not apply to other fields of medicine. In the study of anatomy, comparisons of animal and human structure are taken for granted. The principles of human physiology have been derived largely from experiments made on animals. Studies of the anatomy of the frog, the embryo of the chick, the alimentary functions of the dog, the genetics of the fruit fly, are all integral parts of the study of the human animal. A hormone, crystallized in pure form from the thyroid of sheep, pig, cow or man, may yield the same chemical product and be readily accepted as such. Yet the same behavior responses of man and animal to almost identical situations are difficult for us to accept as illustration of a common principle of psychodynamics. We have accepted our kinship with the animal world structurally and biochemically, but remain isolationist psychologically.

### NATURAL OBSERVATION VERSUS EXPERIMENTATION

Animal psychology became a valid field of scientific study in the latter part of the nineteenth century. Its growth into a scientific discipline involved a long struggle with "nature lovers" and romantic natural historians. It became especially sensitive to all anthropomorphic thinking. The natural historian who mixed together careful observation and careless interpretation was rejected as strongly as the writer of popular books containing a jumble of fact and fable. In the process of liberation from anecdotage, the animal psychologist emulated the experimental biologist and physicist. He narrowed the field of animal studies to precise data verified by measurement and experiment. This purification resulted in a curious situation— that of a discipline in which all knowledge was barred that did not emerge from the laboratory. It might be compared to a field of medicine divested of all clinical knowledge, i.e., knowledge derived from observation and histories of patients at the bedside or in the office. Medical practice would then be limited to the application of that small fraction of medical knowledge which is verified by experiment and by accurate measurement.

Actually, in his day-to-day behavior with animals, the psychologist behaves "clinically" like the physician. He is aware, for example, from his experience with chimpanzees, that one of them appears quite irritable, that another is friendly, that a third is quite likely to make a vicious attack on the experimenter. Moreover, his own behavior to the chimpanzees is based on such knowledge, often with the same assurance, depending on how well he "knows" his animals, as that derived from experimental studies. He depends on the kind of knowledge that goes into the making of human attitudes. His experience teaches him that he has every reason to anticipate the behavior of each chimpanzee in the same manner essentially as he learns to anticipate the behavior of a human being. Yet, for his scientific work, he is loath to study the animal outside the conventional system of observation and controls that comprise the criteria of the experiment.

An event that took place in a center for the study of experimental neurosis in animals may illustrate this point more clearly. An investigator was demonstrating to a class of students the effect of an experimentally produced neurosis on the cardiorespiratory functions of a pig. The animal was prepared in the usual Pavlov frame, and the pulse and respiratory tracings, etc., were made visible to the class. The investigator was about to point out the irregularities in the tracings, as he had done on a number of other occasions. To his surprise, however, the tracings were normal. Proof of the experimental neurosis was not demonstrable.

The mystery was solved very quickly, apparently to

everyone's satisfaction. One of the students present at the time had taken care of the pig during the previous summer season. He became quite fond of the animal and hosed him often during the hot summer days. The pig apparently noticed him among the other students. He grunted in what was interpreted as an affectionate greeting when the student came close. During the next demonstration and thereafter, when the student was no longer present, the pig performed in the anticipated neurotic manner.

It is interesting that this significant event, as important to the psychiatrist as the experiment itself, was not made the basis of an independent investigation. It contained probably the essential ingredients of the "positive transference" of psychoanalysis, and may have aided in a simplification of that concept. Actually, the episode served a purpose in influencing a series of experiments in the center in which it happened. The reactions of a sheep in a Pavlov frame were studied while its lamb was nearby. The study of animal attitudes, in this case compounded of maternal feelings, was thus made secondary to a Pavlovian experiment.

LIMITATIONS OF THEORY AND METHOD

The same episode reveals other restrictions of the animal psychologist. He is often wedded forever to his animal or his instrument. A psychologist who uses the method of Pavlov, for example, feels bound to his apparatus and to the theory of conditioning that seems to be an integral part of it. The apparatus which was first designed to serve the investigator, may in the course of time tend to enslave him. The skill developed in learning to master the new instrument or the theory out of which it evolved may become a controlling interest. The investigator's thoroughness, his erudition which encompasses the literature accumulated by colleagues working with the same device, even his profundity when he is capable of plumbing the depths, may serve finally to restrict his vision. In the extreme instance, the investigator can understand nothing until it passes through the special machinery of his familiar world, translated into his specific language, concepts and methodology. The resistance to new points of view is readily understandable when it involves a modification of technical skills and a system of thinking that represents, besides a lifelong habit, a source of security and self-esteem.

The gradually diminishing returns from the special tool and special theory is a problem that applies to the entire domain of science. It is an important problem, particularly in a young science whose development is easily retarded by rigidities; and in a psychological science whose area is so vast that the temptation always arises of securing a firm foothold, however narrow the field.

### INFLUENCE OF PSYCHOANALYSIS

Animal psychology has had its share of impacts from other disciplines, in recent decades, to shake its complacency with traditional formulae and subject matter. Of the various influences that have widened the scope of animal psychology, most pertinent for psychodynamics is the influence of Freud. This is revealed specifically in the selection of experiments that deal with his theories; generally, in the utilization of psychoanalytic concepts.

The experiments have been concerned with testing hypotheses. Rats, for example, have been used to demonstrate the principle of regression (Mowrer, 1940). When a floor (a steel grill) on which they rested was charged with an electric current, they learned to absorb the shock by sitting on their hind legs. In the next stage of this experiment, the rats learned to turn off the current by pressing a pedal. When this habit was established, it took precedence over the previous habit. That is, whenever the rats felt the electrical shock, they did not sit on their hind legs. Instead, they pressed the pedal which eliminated the painful current entirely. Pressure on the pedal was presumably a superior, as it was also a later, form of adjustment than the earlier one of merely reducing the pain by sitting hunched up in a certain way. The pedal was now charged with electricity. The rats, accustomed to relieve their distress by pressing the pedal, had another shock to contend with. Thereupon, they went back to sitting on their hind legs, their first method of contending with an electrical floor. In other words, according to the experimenter, by surrendering a later and superior method for an earlier and inferior one, they illustrated the principle of regression. The superior method was still available to them, regardless of the charged pedal. A second group of rats, who had never learned the sitting down method, continued to press it even when it became charged, and so cut off the current.

This experiment is a good example of a large number of similar efforts. It may be used as an illustration of the problem involved in the attempt to capture a concept, derived from theorizing about human behavior as it is revealed through free verbalization often vaguely defined, and to pin the concept down to a neat experiment. In the process, the concept is given sharp definition. It is then tested out through the behavior of animals in a controlled situation, so designed that the concept can be translated into activity which belongs exclusively to the concept as

*David M. Levy*

newly defined. The activity which tests the operation of the concept is bound within a framework which it is hoped will demarcate it from the other concepts and so free it from the myriad of relationships with which it was originally perceived in the psychoanalytic situation.

When the experimenter finds that the concept is "valid" he is still at a loss. He wonders if it is the real thing. In the experiment with rats, the investigator called the assumed regression an "analogue" of regression. After all, regression in humans refers to historical regression—a return, in response to a difficulty, to an earlier and inferior mode of adjustment at one time considered appropriate; for example, the return to bed wetting on the part of the older child following the birth of the baby. But is that in principle the behavior of the rat who had learned only two ways of dealing with an electrical floor? Given any two methods of equal or different values, would the rats use the first method if the second were blocked; and if he knew only one method, would he not more likely persist in it, there being nothing else to do? The regressive behavior of the child is one of a variety of possible responses. When the baby comes, if the older child is presumably jealous and feels the loss of love and attention, he may attack it, hit at its crib, talk about it in a derogatory manner, show off, refuse to notice it, or use an opposite tack and show it excessive affection and admiration, etc. Furthermore, the situation in the case of the child is usually said to be a "natural" one; that is, it is the sort of thing that commonly happens. The situation in the case of the rats is "artificial." It is the sort of thing that doesn't happen to rats in their natural state.

The concept of regression, though simpler than most other concepts in psychoanalysis, also remained a problem.

The notion of using an earlier and inferior method of adaptation is simple enough. As a dynamic process, however, it is more difficult to comprehend. Is regression a return to a well-organized mode of behavior, typical of an earlier stage (and also reinforced by "fixation" through erotic determinants according to the original definition), or is it a disorganization? In the supposed regressive behavior of some schizophrenics, investigators have found no evidence of a throwback behavior, since all evidence of the behavior manifested was never previously observed. Is disorganization that has the appearance of regressive behavior to be differentiated from true regression? Also, is it fair to apply the term regression to a previous mode of behavior that has nothing to do with erotic elements?

The experimenter was well aware of the conceptual difficulties in his experiments with rats. Yet, like so many others, he preferred to use a device which was a poor fit for the concept he tried to test. There are numerous examples of regressive behavior in animals to be observed clinically, as in humans. They appear to be identical modes of response. Actually the situation of the older child and the new baby is repeated time and again with the pet dog and the new baby. The most recent example that comes to mind is the return to wetting the floor on the part of a well-trained dachshund when a baby was adopted. The dog displayed the usual repertoire of responses observed on such occasions. He growled at the baby, though he never attacked it; he barked more than usual; he showed off his few tricks repeatedly; he tugged at his mistress' skirts when she fondled the baby. He went through such capers for about six weeks and thereafter "accepted" the situation.

A second example of regressive behavior in a dog was brought to my attention recently. A police dog, the pet of a married couple, was two years old when he was taken in by master and mistress. At the time, the acceptance of this dog was thought to be a risky procedure. The dog was a wanderer, had bitten people, and in an accident had broken his leg. The fracture had been repaired, though at the time when first seen by the present owners, he was still limping. The prospective master and mistress were interested in seeing the animal regardless of his history, because they had always had a police dog and felt that they understood them. They were not disconcerted even by the fact that the dog had been condemned. When they first came to the home of a friend to look over the animal, he showed immediate evidence of affection for one of the prospective owners. It was decided to take him on for a trial period. Within six weeks, the dog gave up his wandering and yelping and biting, and he became an affectionate and docile animal. Ten months after they had the dog in their possession, they had a baby, their first child. There was, of course, some apprehension as to how the dog would take to the baby. When this was tested out, the dog was affectionate to it, certainly showed no evidence of hostility. After a while there was no apprehension about it. Meanwhile, however, a change was noted in the behavior of the animal. He had become less energetic, generally less responsive—he seemed sad.

When the baby was five months old, it was put in a play pen on the floor and given a number of rubber toys. On that day the dog developed a limp. He walked the way he had after the fracture was partially healed. A number of examinations by a veterinarian were made, and the limp was diagnosed as psychic. In a human, no doubt, we would have called it hysterical paralysis. Concerned about the limp and the general listlessness of the animal, the master playfully threw a ball at the dog in the room in which the baby's pen was placed. The dog limped over to the pen and looked at the toys. That gave the master his clue. He bought a number of new rubber toys for the dog, dumped them in front of him, and played ball with him. The dog was apparently quite excited and ran around the room, losing the limp. He had been limping for about three weeks. Evidently the cure was a successful one, since he has never limped since that time, which was over two and a half years ago.

Systematic clinical studies of animal behavior, besides adding to our knowledge, would render superfluous a number of animal experiments designed to discover mechanisms (or "test the claims" of psychoanalysis) readily discerned through observation of spontaneous behavior. Such studies would aid also experimental procedures by indicating those areas in which controlled observations would be most necessary and fruitful.

### SPECIAL ADVANTAGE OF EXPERIMENTAL AS COMPARED WITH CLINICAL STUDIES

Examples of the manner in which the experiment aids the clinical investigator may be cited. The first is concerned with the influence of special events in infancy on adult behavior. In this experiment a number of rats were subjected to periods of hunger in infancy. To test the effect of this experience in adult life, the amount of food they hoarded was measured. Some of the rats who had experienced the state of hunger in infancy hoarded much more than the others.

The investigator stated that his experiment was devised in order to get controlled evidence concerning the claims

David M. Levy

of psychoanalysis that experiences during infancy can affect adult behavior (Hunt, 1941). Such claims are shared by psychiatrists generally, child psychologists, educators, and a variety of investigators in other disciplines. They are easily verified by the study of case records in any number of schools and clinics. In one sense, therefore, like the previous experiment, an attempt was made to verify the obvious. Further, the main line of sequence—infantile starvation— increased adult hoarding—is not necessarily a test of the claims "that experiences during infancy affect adult behavior." Suppose there were no difference in regard to adult hoarding among the control and experimental rats. One could then conclude only that the experience of starvation in the infancy of the rats was not followed by a particular type of behavior (hoarding) in adult life.

The experiment was selected for this lecture, not as verification, but as an illustration of its particular advantage over clinical studies. The starvation period can be controlled. You can place it any day you wish. You can starve the rat much or little. You can control various aspects of the experience in a manner which renders your conclusions more definite, sure and accessible than those derived from untangling a pattern out of the web of human behavior.

The experience of starvation, though equal in terms of diminution of food and span of time, was initiated at different ages. It was started in one group of infant rats when they were twenty-four days old, and in another when they were thirty-two days old. Only the twenty-four-day group manifested excessive hoarding. The thirty-two-day group hoarded no more than the controls. Evidently, response to the particular experience of starvation was significantly altered by a difference of eight days of age.

To test differences in hoarding in adult life, all the animals, experimental and control, were subjected to a preliminary period of partial starvation. They were given just enough food for subsistence for five days, in order to stimulate them to collect the pellets of food, the number of which constituted the measure of hoarding. The preliminary period of starvation was necessary because rats who are well fed have little or no propensity to hoard.

The experiment offers a good illustration of "operational" value. The starvation period can be produced at any time in the life of the animal, so that the period of susceptibility in infancy can be accurately determined. We know in the group of animals studied that, in terms of hoarding, starvation must be experienced before thirty-two days of age to have an effect in adult life. But how severe must the starvation be? The experimental tool allows a measure of the experience in terms of food privation applied as a single experience, or as one of a series, or in a variety of combinations. What is the minimal experience of starvation that will have an effect on adult hoarding at the most susceptible age? How severe must the experience be at the least susceptible age to have an effect? There is involved the problem of susceptibility in terms also of individual differences of personality. That would require, besides genetic studies, the kind of clinical observations that are made in humans.

There remains the large variety of "traumata" to be studied in the same manner as starvation. The investigator referred to observations that thirst alone, as well as hunger, was followed by an increase in hoarding. Would fear-provoking experiences in infancy or later have a similar effect? Is hoarding a general rather than a specific tension-

*David M. Levy*

relieving outlet? We know that it is rendered excessive by more than one type of experience.

PSYCHOLOGICAL VULNERABILITY

The points raised in the previous paragraph indicate the special advantage of experimental procedures over clinical observations in the solution of problems requiring precise control. Their application to problems in human behavior is quite direct. The evaluation of a disturbing event in infancy on the individual personality requires, besides knowledge of particulars, knowledge also of general laws of special susceptibility in terms of developmental age and of the type of external agent. What difference does it make if event A (a fright, a period of separation from the mother, a change to a new place of residence, or an experience of starvation) occurs when a child is age three months, nine months, two years, three years? Holding the age factor constant, what difference does the type of experience make? It is in this area that so much of value can be learned for preventive psychiatry.

Case studies carefully compiled furnish details that may approximate an experimental situation. It has been found, for example, that presumably normal children who undergo surgical procedures when aged twelve to twenty-four months are much more likely to have subsequent emotional difficulties than when operated on after that age. It has been found also that the twelve- to twenty-four-month group manifest such difficulties in the form of rather uncomplicated anxiety symptoms (fears, phobias, and increased dependency) as compared with older groups, whose anxieties when they occur are more likely to be complicated by aggressive behavior. The age factor (twelve to twenty-four months) appears to be more significant than any other factor investigated (dependency on the mother, special experiences, etc.). In terms of available data, susceptibility is very high in the second year of life (involving the majority of children at that age), fairly high in the third year of life (involving a third), and of decreasing magnitude in later years. Similar studies for the first year of life are not at hand.

The special vulnerability of the organism to a variety of disturbances of function, emotional and physiological, may follow the same general principle in a number of animal species. Each type of disturbance may have its own particular mode of function, aside from the individual unique response. But the uniqueness of response requires full study. However emotionally vulnerable to an operation an infant may be at eighteen months, a study of his response to that procedure cannot be understood as an individual experience without knowledge of his personality, which includes all his typical modes of behavior, and also the specific history of his emotional growth. The same applies to animals.

The specific influence of psychoanalysis on animal psychology has been illustrated in two sets of experiments. In the first, the main difficulty for the experimenter was to place the animal in a situation comparable to one in humans. In the second, the difficulty was easily solved since the task was simply to prove that an event in infancy has an effect in adult life, and was therefore readily applicable to animals. On the whole, psychoanalysis has had more influence on the concepts of the animal psychologist than on his specific experiments. This influence bears fruit eventually in experimentation, but the direct connection with the psychoanalytic concept, out of which the experiment

*David M. Levy*

emerged, is often lost and may even be unknown to the investigator. A large number of experiments in frustration, for example, though initiated by psychoanalytic concepts, have, in the course of time, become imbedded in the method and the language of the experimenter, and regarded as an offshoot of findings originating in the laboratory. The psychoanalyst who reads the literature and listens to papers by experimental animal psychologists, even by those apparently opposed to psychoanalytic concepts or unaware of them, meets many familiar Freudian ideas. They are seen particularly in experiments and discussions of drives, needs, goals, motivation, conflict, frustration, shame, anxiety, sex, aggression and regression.

### EXPERIMENTAL NEUROSIS

The field of activity in animal psychology most directly related to psychopathology owes its origin to Pavlov (1927). He observed various mental states of immobility in dogs that were by-products, so to speak, of salivary conditioning experiments. An accident was probably more effective than any other factor in stimulating the experimenter's interest in the animal's abnormal mental states. Pavlov's dogs were subjected to a severe experiment, unaccounted for in the series listed in the laboratory notebooks. Their kennels were suddenly submerged by a rapidly rising flood. During their exhausting struggles to escape drowning by swimming in trapped space, there were flashes of lightning and a variety of explosive sounds near and far—rushing water, falling timber, claps of thunder. For some months after their rescue, they showed, besides the effects of exhaustion, generally depressive states and abnormal reflexes of the kind now made so familiar to us in the numerous studies of "experimental neurosis." Though the dogs recovered in time from their state of shock and became to all outward appearance as normal as they had been before, when one of them was tested by the sight of a trickle of water flowing under a door, the acute anxiety state followed immediately.

Reproduction of abnormal mental states was accomplished in the experimental situation by repeatedly imposing a task on the dog beyond his power of discrimination. The abnormal emotional states which resulted were measured in the usual Pavlovian manner, through their physiological expression in pulse frequency, blood pressure, salivary flow, etc. Not all dogs can be made "neurotic" by the methods employed. Though a constitutional difference may be taken for granted, there is still much to be learned about the significance of the experience for the individual animal. Liddell (1942) has indicated a number of the difficulties involved. He states that the setting in which conditioning experiments ordinarily take place is itself a traumatic situation. The animal is in a state of tension no matter how simple the task, because of the degree of restraint involved in controlling its movement and withstanding the monotony of repeated stimuli, as long as the experiment goes on. The animal's relation to the experimenter, Liddell states, must also be considered. Let us assume that the dog's relationship to the experimenter is such that he is very eager to succeed in performing his task. He is then, theoretically, more likely to develop an experimental neurosis, because he will more likely persist in attempting a discrimination that is beyond him. The reverse would also follow. The less "goal-directed," the less likely will the dog be caught in the trap of straining all efforts to do the impossible. Why does the experiment have to be repeated a number of times to produce the neurosis? Because the animal presumably is able to dissipate the effects in some manner, most likely by releasing pent-up energy through running about and sleeping it off. If the interval of time between the experiment is too long, the neurosis does not take place. Hence, the repetitions must be so placed in time that the dog's own curative functions are not allowed to go on to completion. The process is thus analogous to accumulation of tensions in a person who can hardly overcome the emotional effects of one crisis before he finds himself in another and then another, until he breaks down.

The experimental neurosis as conceived by Pavlov may be regarded as a functional disturbance originating in the cortex of an animal, strongly goal-directed, probably constitutionally predisposed, and in a situation involving physical and emotional strain. Pavlov was interested primarily in the instrument of discrimination, the cortex as a mechanism, rather than in the animal as a motivated organism. The experiment is not analogous to the flood, whether one accepts or rejects the theory that the focus of the disturbance in the former lies in the problem of discriminating two closely matched stimuli. In the flood there was no problem of that sort. There was no need to discriminate. There was one obvious danger and a desperate attempt to escape it. Furthermore, the escape was successful. The animals were saved and recovered their ability to respond to conditioning experiments. True, a reminder of the experience —the sight of water dripping under the door—precipitated anxiety. The anxiety remained latent. It was not manifested in the experiment after recovery. Unlike the experimental neurosis which produces a more or less chronic and generalized dysfunction, the experience of the flood operated to produce anxiety only when a sample of the original event (that operated quite like a "symbol") was brought to the consciousness of the animal. In contrast with the experimental neurosis, which is analogous to schizophrenia, the experience of the flood resulted in a phobia.

### CLINICAL NEUROSIS AND PSYCHOPATHOLOGY

Generally, in animals as in humans, one fear-provoking or painful experience may carry potent reminders for a long time. The monkey who coughed and spluttered and ran when a lighted cigarette was brought near his nose, acted the same way later when a piece of cigarette paper was brought near. A hen, once frightened by the sight of a guinea pig, always avoided the room in which the event occurred, in spite of inducements of heaps of grain. The locality of a disturbing event has particular significance. The place where danger threatens evidently must be well remembered if the animal is to survive. Response to the single threatening event, often so excessively traumatic to the human psyche, is well revealed as a basic adaptation in animal studies.

The biologist, Whitman (1899), made an interesting experiment and an interesting deduction relating to this subject. During the mother bird's absence, he displaced one of her eggs, putting it on the rim of her nest. In the case of the robin there was immediate abandonment. In the case of the pigeon, there was quite a different response. The pigeon worked the egg back to its original position and continued its brooding. The robin's response was an immediate instinctive reaction to change in a familiar visual configuration. A wild bird must act in stereotyped fashion. The locus of its nest, its structure, its relation to the immediate environment, is selected with an eye to safety. The

*61*

bird is alerted to every detail of its habitat. The slightest alteration is a danger signal. There is no time to investigate. The solution is flight. Unlike the robin, the pigeon was domesticated. Its sense of danger was lulled. Safety means time and opportunity for selection. The pigeon could afford the time for more learning, for more plasticity, therefore, of instinctive behavior. How Whitman's observations hold for all bird species, I do not know, but the principle that modifiability of "instinctive" behavior is facilitated by security and diminished by danger, though not absolute, appears to be well founded. That it applies to a response as fundamental as reaction to a site of danger indicates that many "innate" responses are plastic. Memory of place applies also to pleasurable and exciting experiences. The memory of safety areas is also important for survival. The significance of such place memories in human psychology is well illustrated in clinical histories, often strikingly in dreams.

In relation to the psychoses, animal psychology has furnished chiefly "analogues" of hypnosis, catalepsy, catatonia. Thus far they have contributed little to our understanding of psychotic states.

Reactive depressions in animals appear to be of a different order (Tinkelpaugh, 1928). They are not "analogues." They contain essentially the same type of depressive response to the loss of a loved object as we observe in humans. The mourning of a dog for his departed master is a familiar example. The story of Cupid, a young Rhesus monkey, has become a classic example of emotional turmoil arising out of "marital" difficulties. The response finally took the form of an agitated depression. The account contains all the elements of conflict, guilt, privation, devotion, masochism and love. Cupid was first attached to an older female with whom he lived monogamously for three years. She was then taken away. A simple depression ensued. He was given a young female to whom he adjusted after an initial period of hostility. Some time after the new relationship had been established, apparently with success, he was led past the cage of his first female. Their eyes met. She shrieked excitedly. Cupid's psychosis followed immediately. He bit himself repeatedly and severely, causing deep lacerations. He became restless and agitated. He would not eat. He withdrew all contact from his second female and his human attendants. After some time, the psychologist restored the first mate. The change was favorable. The older female fondled Cupid, nursed him devotedly, and gradually "calmed his nerves." Fourteen months elapsed before he recovered.

The organic and toxic psychoses of animals, though similar in their essential pathology to those of humans, have not been investigated from the point of view of psychodynamics. The variations in the response of dogs to hydrophobia, of horses to locoweed, of cattle to snakeroot, etc., have not been explored, except as symptoms of brain pathology.

Mental deficiencies occur in animals as well as in men and can be classified according to etiology in the same manner; for example, developmental defects, prenatal infections, inherited amentia, etc. Mentally defective animals have been studied almost exclusively in zoos. Presumably they do not survive in a state of nature.

### SOME BASIC STUDIES IN PSYCHODYNAMICS

For the rest, I propose to list a number of basic studies in psychodynamics, in which the investigation of animal behavior may play an essential role, or indeed might have

*David M. Levy*

done so already if we had integrated available knowledge. The list proposed is not intended to cover the field. It includes examples derived partly out of my own attempts to solve problems arising in psychiatric work with children by means of animal studies; and partly out of ideas that stem from current interests and discussions with colleagues in psychoanalysis and animal psychology.

### a. Primary Needs

Among primary needs are included all innate needs of the organism, whatever function they subserve—chemical, physiological, emotional, social, etc.

An example of a chemical need is the need of calcium. Hens deprived of calcium appear to go on a frantic search for it. They will peck at buttons and other hard objects. When supplied with calcium after being starved of it, they will eat about the same amount, whether it is exposed to their view or concealed in other food. How do they know what they need? How do they know when their need is satisfied?

These problems have not been solved, but the theories which represent tentative answers, and the lines of inquiry apply to humans as well as animals. In a state of tension arising from a chemical dysbalance, the animal is restless and searches in a manner that appears to be somewhat guided. When the appropriate food is found, it is ingested until the animal is "satisfied"; in other words, until the internal environment is in equilibrium. The release of tension is concomitant with the inner chemical balance.

The usual need of food is felt specifically as hunger, and the physiological gastric mechanism that first initiates the feeling has been thoroughly investigated. The need of cal-

64

cium and other special mineral foods or hormones is not felt specifically like hunger or thirst. It is felt more vaguely as discomfort, or restlessness, or a general anxious state.

Sucking is apparently an innate physiological need (Levy, 1934a). The mammalian fetus has been exercising mouth and neck muscles repeatedly in preparation for sucking and swallowing. As in the case of many other needs, once the process of satisfying a sucking need is initiated, it goes on to a point of satiety, of fulfillment. If that point is not reached when a feeding is finished at breast or bottle, the lips remain tense. Babies or puppies who have been deprived of sucking activity too soon can sometimes be observed making sucking movements after breast or bottle has been withdrawn. When the sucking phase of the feeding act in repeated feedings remains incomplete, then finger sucking or some other substitute form of sucking is bound to follow.

A recent clinical study was made of the average daily sucking time of thirty babies, each age seven months. The group contained fifteen babies who were finger suckers and fifteen who had never developed that habit. When the average number of minutes of sucking time per day for each of the thirty infants was arranged from high to low, not one case of finger sucking occurred at the high end of the scale (130 or more). Every infant whose average time was at the low end of the scale (70 or less) was a finger sucker.

The relation of diminished sucking time and substitute sucking activities has been verified experimentally in dogs. Observations of calves, kittens and monkeys show similar findings.

The need of pecking in chickens illustrates the same principle as the need of sucking. Chicks reared on a wire floor, with the same amount of food available as an adjoining control group, develop the habit of feather pulling. Chicks who are on the wire have no opportunity to satisfy their pecking needs on the wooden floor of the hen house or on the ground (Levy, 1934b).

Body movement is another functional need that follows the general pattern of physiologic needs in terms of periodicity, cyclic curve of energy discharge, end point, and specific evidence of incompleteness (Levy, 1944). In a number of vertebrate species, it has been found that when the animal is confined for a long period of time in a space too small to allow locomotion, it develops head tics (e.g., weaving tic of horses, head tic of bears, head shakes of chickens). Similar head tics have been observed in infants confined too long in cribs.

When space is inadequate to satisfy movement need but large enough to allow locomotion (as in cages at the zoo) stereotyped movements develop. The result of restraint of movement for short periods of time is a temporary movement excess, as in dogs who are released after a period of restraint at the leash, or children at recess after a period of restraint in the classroom. Observations of an infant in the creeping stage and later in the walking stage, who was confined in a playpen all day except for two periods of forty-five minutes, revealed excessive motor activity during the intervals of free movement.

The physiological needs are closely related to developmental age. The need of body movement, for example, is greater in the second half year of life than in the first. The needs increase in their early stages with successive fulfillments. Thus, the need of movement is greater after a child has experienced freedom of movement.

It may follow also that restraint of a need before it has

attained fulfillment (as, for example, in the continuous restraint of American Indian babies in the cradle board) may diminish a need. In the case of the pecking need, when chicks are prevented from fulfilling it and are fed from a dropper the first two weeks of life, the need is lost. Without prolonged efforts on the part of the psychologist to restore it, the chicks would die (Bird, 1933). Needs cannot survive *in vacuo*. The outer and inner environments are concomitant parts of their function.

Each need has its own history, its peculiar pattern, its range of modifiability. Each requires special investigation.

Emotional needs have not been studied in animals as thoroughly as physiological needs, for the reason that they are usually not regarded as primary needs. In the animal's attempt to initiate and complete the act that represents the operation of a need, emotional factors are considered as an integral part of the process at every stage. The need of a feeling, however—as a more or less specific source of tension and striving—is difficult to comprehend as clearly as the more tangible concept of a need of food or sex. In the category of needs, the need of sex is envisaged primarily as a physiological need, however deflected, diminished, or exaggerated it may become through emotional influence. The feeling appropriate to the need of sex, like the need of food, involves specific physiological activity. The animal's need of social relationship, if such a need exists in primary form, as implied in the concepts of social or herd instinct, would be an example of a primary emotional need. The need of maternal love, as a primary emotional need, has been studied clinically in children. Case studies of children deprived of maternal love, though not deprived of the usual nursing care, protection and training, reveal specific personality difficulties. They include symptoms of "primary affect hunger" (Levy, 1937)—basically an excessive craving for love through close personal relationships, with derivative symptoms, and in a smaller number of cases an apparent loss or diminution of the need for love with resultant lack of response to emotional influence (the "deprived psychopath"). Emotional ties appear to be a primary need and probably a basic component of other needs involving mutual relationships—sexual, maternal, or social. The need for love appears also to follow the law of certain physiologic needs in regard to excess and diminution.

Experiments on emotional needs of animals have hardly begun. They would reach the core of this problem more successfully than clinical studies. The case of an emotionally deprived dog has been cited in the literature (Levy, 1942/43).

### b. Maternal Drive

In the maternal activities of birds and mammals, including humans, the same basic factors are manifest: namely, contact (warmth), care (feeding, cleaning), protection, and training. The maternal drive, as measured in animals, is stronger than thirst, hunger, or sex. In experimental studies of the strength of drives, the barrier that had to be crossed to attain the goal to which the drive was erected was an electrified grill with a measurable charge (Warden, 1931). How humans would respond to a similar experiment is not known, though it would seem safe to conclude from clinical data that in a certain percentage of mothers the results would be the same. There is evidently a range in the strength of the maternal drive, a normal distribution curve, in humans as in animals (Wiesner and Sheard, 1933).

## c. *Aggression and Domination*

The classical research on the peck order in chickens was followed by a series of investigations which demonstrated a general principle of domination among vertebrates (Schjelderup-Ebbe, 1922). The peck order, the rule whereby a rigid caste system develops in a community of animals (so that animal A always maintains ascendancy over animal B, animal B over animal C, and so on down the line) is not inflexible. There are many variations of the original formula, though the principle remains. In a barnyard of sixty hens who have lived together for several months, every hen knows exactly who is above it and who is below it. However this type of social organization has come about, it makes for a more static, stable, and apparently advantageous adjustment.

When two monkeys, strangers to each other, are put together in a cage, one becomes boss over the other, often in a minute's time. They size each other up. It is literally size that usually determines the result, though strength, agility, persistence or bluff in any of their combinations may determine the outcome (Maslow, 1940).

The dominating tendency of human beings, as an innate biosocial response, requires further exploration in the light of these studies. Our usual explanations of aggressive domination in humans are in terms of competitive strivings for maternal love (as in sibling rivalry); compensatory aggression because of anticipated rebuff or anticipated unconscious accusations in social relationships; compensatory aggression based on feelings of inadequacy; as a reaction against submissive, dependent attitudes, etc. They may be appropriate to the data of a given case, yet fail to take into consideration what may prove to be basic biological drives.

*David M. Levy*

Analogous to the behavior of animals is our own "sizing up" of a new acquaintance and that large variety of human reactions to the stranger—boys ganging up on a newcomer, the primitive's fear of witchcraft in the neighboring village, the suspicion or even the tentative or ceremonious approach to the new neighbor.

The hens' reaction to a strange hen, even one of their own breed, is to attack it after a minute or two of "sizing it up." The newcomer's personality changes under one's eyes within a short time. Regardless of her previous relationship to other hens, she becomes an outcast. She avoids all places in the henhouse where hens are crowded together. She keeps away from the trough and pecks from the floor. She appears furtive and apprehensive. She keeps isolated from the others. She walks slowly or makes sudden runs as though always in danger. The fury of pecks in her first half hour of the new residence gradually subsides. Within ten days to two weeks she appears "blended"; it is hard to tell her behavior from the rest.

Little chicks are friendly. The strange chick isn't pecked, though for a while it avoids the others and tries desperately to get back home. At about six weeks of age, the chicks act like the grownups and attack strange chicks very quickly.

The reaction appears to be an innate response of anxiety in the presence of the unfamiliar that comes after a period of maturation, followed—in the case of unfamiliar chicks —by an attack.

Aggression in animals as in humans is capable of a high degree of modification and a large variety of manifestations. A wounded dog, treated by its master, may visibly curb its "reflex" tendency to bite when its painful leg is moved. As in humans also, a dog may express its frustration through release of aggression. One of my dogs, up to his sixth or seventh year of life, would bite at a bush when I would refuse to throw a ball for him to fetch. Thereafter, his response to the same type of frustrating situation was patient waiting or insistent barking. Some animals have modified their aggression more successfully than man. The howler monkeys, for example, hardly ever assault each other. Their aggression takes the form of vocalization.

Dominant behavior, as an attempt to satisfy a need for social status, has been so interpreted in chimpanzees and other animals (Yerkes, 1943).

### d. *Aggression and Sex*

Though all drives require some form of aggression to fulfill their object (using the term "aggression" to include all varieties of self-assertive behavior), a higher magnitude is required whenever the drive involves the play of an ascendant role. The sexual drive, in its relation to social ascendancy and submission, is clearly depicted in a number of animal studies. Among chimpanzees, for example, it appears that the female, when highly aggressive as compared with her mate, limits her period of copulation to her few days of ovulation. When submissive to her mate, she yields to his sex demands all through the menstrual cycle including the period of bleeding. When females are ascendant in the scale of domination, they may appear to struggle against surrender to their own sexual needs, because sexual submission to the male may be followed by loss of a dominant position previously held over him (Yerkes, 1943).

Many animals utilize sexual activity at times as an act of sheer dominance.

*71*

*David M. Levy*

*e. Negativism*

The period of human infancy, starting around fifteen to eighteen months of age and proceeding to about four and a half years of age, has been called the first adolescence. Indeed, the resemblance to the age of puberty is quite striking. The "striving for independence," the "I'll do it myself" of the first adolescence, is frequently manifested in negativistic behavior (as also in the puberty adolescence). Animals may show similar transformation when they grow beyond the earliest dependency period. Resistant or negativistic behavior appears to be a protective barrier against excessive demands on the organism, a protection also against superior force. It is used also as a weapon of hostility, in the form of spite, revenge, and domination. Negativistic phenomena are seen in psychiatry as "normal" stubbornness, as compulsive behavior, and in its extreme form, as manifestations of catatonia. Various forms of repetitive behavior, the "fixated responses" of animals, belong to this category.

In certain experiments in which rats had learned to jump over a barrier to butt their way through the correct one of two hard paper doors which swung open onto a cubicle containing food, both doors were fixed so that all ensuing efforts were unsuccessful (Maier, 1946; Maier and Klee, 1941). Whichever door the rats tried to enter, and they were forced to make the jumps, they were "frustrated." Under these conditions a variety of reactions occurred, including "a fixed reaction" in a certain small percentage of the animals. Within the "fixated" group, for example, some rats would jump only to the right door and never to the left, even after the left door was later opened and the food in that cubicle exposed. Such fixed reactions

72

may have a basic element in common with a number of compulsive negativistic reactions of humans.

Our relation to the other mammals is seen not only as anatomical and physiological; it is seen also in psychological studies and includes the basic drives. These examples of animal experiments that illuminate the domain of human behavior represent a small selection out of many. They have served their purpose well if they have helped you to recognize the fact that we are linked to the animal species by psychological as well as biological ties.

## REFERENCES

Allee, W. C. (1938), *The Social Life of Animals*. New York: Norton.

Beach, Frank A. (1947), *Hormones and Behavior*. New York: Paul B. Hoeber.

Brückner, G. H. Untersuchungen zur Tiersoziologie, insbesondere zur Auflösung der Familie, *Ztschr. Psychol., 128*: 1-110, 1933.

Bird, C. (1933), Maturation and Practices: Their Effects Upon the Feeding Reaction of Chicks. *J. Comparat. Psychol., 16*: 343.

Carpenter, C. R. (1934), A Field Study of the Behavior and Social Relations of Howling Monkeys. *Comparat. Psychol. Monographs, 10*.

Collias, U. (1944), Aggressive Behavior Among Vertebrate Animals. *J. Physiol. Zool., 17*:83-123.

Darling, F. Frazer (1937), *A Herd of Red Deer*. London: Oxford University Press.

Gantt, W. H. (1944), *Experimental Basis for Neurotic Behavior*. New York: Paul B. Hoeber.

Hunt, J. McV. (1941), The Effects of Infant Feeding-Frustration upon Adult Hoarding in the Albino Rat. *J. Abn. & Soc. Psychol., 36*:338-361.

David M. Levy

Katz, David (1937), *Animals and Men*. New York: Longmans, Green.

Kellogg and Kellogg (1933), *The Ape and the Child*. New York: McGraw-Hill.

Köhler, W. (1925), *The Mentality of Apes*. New York: Harcourt, Brace.

Levy, David M. (1934a), Experiments on the Sucking Reflex and Social Behavior of Dogs. *Am. J. Orthopsychiat*, 4:203-224.

—— (1934b), On Instinct Satiation: An Experiment on the Pecking Behavior of Chickens. *J. Gen. Psychol.*, 18:327-348 or, A Note on Pecking in Chickens. *Psychoanal. Quart.* 4:612-613.

—— (1937), Primary Affect Hunger. *Am. J. Psychiat.*, 94:643-652.

—— (1942/43), Psychopathic Personality and Crime. *J. Ed. Sociol.*, 16:99-114.

—— (1944), On the Problem of Movement Restraint. *Am. J. Orthopsychiat.*, 14:644-671.

—— (1945), Psychic Trauma of Operations in Children. *Am. J. Dis. Children*, 69:7-25.

Liddell, H. S. (1942), The Instinctual Processes Through the Influence of Conditioned Reflexes. *Psychosom. Med.*, 4:390-395.

Maier, N. R. F. (1946), Abnormal Fixations. *Am. Psychol.*, 1:462. Abstract.

Maier, N. R. F. and Klee, J. B. (1941), Studies of Abnormal Behavior in the Rat, VII. *J. Exp. Psychol.*, 29:380-389.

Maslow, A. H. (1940), Dominance-Quality and Social Behavior in Infra-Human Primates. *J. Soc. Psychol.*, 11:313-324.

Masserman, J. H. (1942), Psychological Dynamism in Behavior. *Psychiatry*, 5:341-348.

Moss, F. A. Ed. (1946), *Comparative Psychology*. New York: Prentice-Hall.

Mowrer, O. H. (1940), An Experimental Analogue of "Regression" with Incidental Observations on "Reaction Formation." *J. Abn. & Soc. Psychol.*, 35:56-87.

Noble, R. C. (1945), *The Nature of the Beast*. New York: Doubleday.

Animal Psychology and Psychiatry

Pavlov, I. P. (1927), *Conditioned Reflexes*. London: Oxford University Press.

Schjelderup-Ebbe, J. (1922), Beiträge zur Soziolpsychologie des Haushuhns. *Ztschr. Psychol., 88*:225-232.

Tinkelpaugh, O. L. (1928), The Self-Mutilation of a Male Macacus Rhesus Monkey. *J. Mammalogy, 9*:293-300.

Warden, C. J. (1931), *Animal Motivations: Experimental Studies in the Albino Rat*. New York: Columbia University Press.

Whitman, Charles O. (1899), Biological Lectures, 1898; from the Marine Biological Laboratory, Woods Hole, Mass. Boston.

Wiesner, B. P. and Sheard, N. M. (1933), *Maternal Behavior in the Rat*. London: Oliver & Boyd.

Yerkes, R. M. (1943), *Chimpanzees*. New Haven: Yale University Press.

Zuckerman, S. (1932), *The Social Life of Monkeys and Apes*. New York: Harcourt, Brace.

# QUEST FOR ANTIBIOTICS

## By Paul R. Burkholder, Ph. D.

FOR millions of men and women living at the mid twentieth century period, antibiotics represent the ultramodern attainment in practical biology and medicine. The new antibiotic drugs work like magic against many of mankind's old diseases which down through the ages were incurable and fatal. One can read behind the simple tombstone records of life and death in the preceding centuries how, without the numerous benefits of modern medicine, the young were commonly cut off with no chance to live long, productive, and happy lives.

In telling the story of antibiotic investigations in the laboratory and the relation of such scientific discoveries to the welfare of mankind, it is hoped that the audience may learn to appreciate better the significance of basic research in the development of fundamental knowledge which has made possible such fruitful applications in conserving health and lengthening the span of human lives. We shall discuss here what antibiotics are, where they come from and how they are studied. With simple techniques it can be shown that antibiotics probably exist almost everywhere around us and participate in important ways to help preserve the balance of nature. It is remarkable, indeed, that only recently have men of science approached toward an understanding of the powerful effects of these antibiotics and through good fortune have envisioned ways by which the people shall not perish.

## WHAT ARE ANTIBIOTICS?

Antibiotic substances are chemical compounds derived from, or produced by, living organisms, which can in small amounts inhibit the life processes of other organisms. It is relatively unimportant whether the organism producing an antibiotic substance is a macro- or microorganism; some large trees and many very small bacteria can form antibiotic products in their metabolic processes. Such powerful organic substances, which antagonize the growth and possibly prevent the survival of susceptible organisms, may sometimes be prepared by chemical synthesis in the laboratory. Their effectiveness at comparatively low concentrations suggests that antibiotics may function by checking certain especially important enzymatic processes in the inhibited cells. Some antibiotics are poisonous to many kinds of organisms, while others prevent growth of only a few selected kinds of bacteria. Those persons who are concerned with the uses of antibiotics in treating diseases are primarily interested in substances which in low concentrations prevent growth of pathogenic microorganisms, and at the same time show no toxic manifestations in animals and man or do not harm crop plants. Only a few antibiotics have thus far become important drugs for veterinary and human use, and no large-scale application of antibiotics has yet been found in crop protection. Here much work remains to be done; indeed, the task has only just been started.

*Paul R. Burkholder*

Although the word "antibiotic," coined by Vuillemin in 1889, has a very broad meaning as an agent "against life," still the major significance of the term has been developed in the field of antibiotic microbiology. The concept of antibiosis is easily open to misinterpretation. Because of its inherent activity against some forms of life, one must not conclude that an antibiotic substance is active against all life. A therapeutic agent which inhibits certain disease germs may obviously become instrumental in saving the lives of many people. The point which should be emphasized here is that antibiotic substances are generally selective in their antimicrobial activity, and that for application to particular human interests the special properties of any compound must be well understood.

WHERE ARE ANTIBIOTICS FOUND?

Studies on the microorganisms which occur throughout the soils of the world, in decaying organic materials and in natural waters, have demonstrated that characteristic types of bacteria, fungi, protozoa, and other microbes live in great numbers in habitats which are well suited to their requirements. One very striking fact is that pathogenic microorganisms generally do not multipy and grow abundantly in the soils and waters of the earth. Extensive surveys of the occurrence of antibiotic-producing organisms in most of the countries of the world indicate that cultures of bacteria, molds and actinomycetes, producing antimicrobial substances, can be found almost everywhere. In our antibiotic program at Yale, tens of thousands of actinomycete isolations have been made from various geographic regions, such as Egypt, Palestine, Jamaica, California, and Baffin Land. Antibiotic "actinos" are widely distributed,

*78*

occurring in noticeable abundance in the relatively arid grasslands of the world.

In our own experience it has been found that about half of the actinomycetes and the lichen species possess antibiotic properties. The occurrence of antibiosis in molds has been emphasized by the discovery of penicillin by Alexander Fleming in 1928, and since that time many other substances have been isolated from this group. Among the higher fungi also, numerous examples of compounds active against various bacteria have been found. Large groups of higher plants, too, have been surveyed in several laboratories recently and many substances of plant origin are now known to inhibit molds and bacteria. Possibly the oldest of all therapeutic antibiotics is quinine, obtained from the cinchona tree, so important in combating malaria. It can be said, then, that numerous representatives of the fungi, algae, lichens, and higher plants produce antibiotic substances. Perhaps this is one of the reasons why pathogenic bacteria cannot multiply well in the soil, and do not generally form there a menacing reservoir of disease. Though antibacterial and antifungal substances are produced in soils, it is doubtless true that far greater yields of these compounds can be produced in the laboratory with pure cultures, special substrates, and selected conditions of the environment.

The broad ecological aspects of antibiotics has received attention only recently. Along with the mutually beneficial relationships known to occur among symbiotic species and the parasitic actions of those creatures which live at the expense of their hosts, the antagonistic relations of various components in heterogeneous populations are now recognized as having important implications for the distribution of organisms in time and space. In addition to the phenomena of physiological competition for foodstuffs in nature, one needs to consider also the selective pressure which is exerted in the chemical conflicts among the strong and the weak microbes of natural habitats. In the natural relationships of parasitism and symbiosis, there are transfers or exchanges of metabolic substances among different organisms. These relationships may be harmful or beneficial to some organisms. The inhibitory products of the metabolism of some species may be excreted into the environment, and find their way into other living systems where toxic reactions can result in arrested growth or outright destruction of life. By the scientific application of such chemical agents possessing selective and powerful inhibitory action against the causal agents of human and animal diseases, the undesirable activities of parasites can be alleviated or avoided.

### HOW WERE ANTIBIOTICS DISCOVERED?

From ancient times man has searched for remedies with which to cure his diseases. Unfortunately, most remedies of primitive medicine men failed to effect the desired cures, even though faith in them was not lacking. The folk remedies of many countries and the belief in the medicinal properties of fungi, moldy bread, mosses, sea plants, and mud poultices have been perpetuated for centuries. Any values which these remedies may actually possess became known through trial-and-error methods rather than as a result of any scientific knowledge. A few of the reputed remedies of folk medicine appear in the light of current knowledge to have some basis in the antibiotic properties of the materials used. For example, an interesting early Chinese remedy for tuberculosis appears to have consisted of lichen extracts; and recent research indicates that these lichens possess special antibiotic activity against tuberculosis germs. The anthelminthic drugs, santonin and oil of chenopodium were used in crude plant preparations by ancient civilizations.

Although the history of antibiotics in microbiology indicates that in the latter part of the nineteenth century considerable knowledge had accumulated concerning the inhibitory properties of numerous fungi and bacteria against saprophytic and parasitic types of microorganisms, the biological observations during this period were far superior to the meagre chemical work which was accomplished. As early as 1877 Pasteur and associates described the antagonism between common bacteria and anthrax organisms and expressed their hope that such observations might eventually lead to effective therapeutic practices.

The blue pigment, pyocyanin, which was obtained in crystalline form in 1860 has been acclaimed as the first discovered antibiotic substance of microbial origin. The first illustration of antibiosis is said to be Hoppe-Seyler's photograph of the inhibition of anthrax bacilli by a micrococcus in agar plate experiments performed by Doehle in 1889. The first antibiotic isolated from a fungus is mycophenolic acid prepared in crystalline form by Gosio in 1896. Its antibiotic properties were not discovered until fifty years later.

The development of successful antibiotic drugs from the products of microorganisms needed a new point of view and the combined skills of the microbiologist, chemist, pharmacologist and clinician. A new viewpoint was created by research published from several different laboratories in the period from 1936 to 1940. The isolation of gliotoxin in 1936 by Weindling from cultures of *Gliocladium fimbria-*

*Paul R. Burkholder*

*tum* and its recognition as a fungistatic compound is one of the most important contributions to the whole field of antibiotics. A series of remarkable investigations by Dubos (1939) on the tryothricin complex produced by certain Gram-positive spore-forming bacteria drew attention to an important source of antibacterial substances. The phenomenon studied by Dubos and his colleagues was not different from that which engaged the attention of Duclaux some forty years before, but the isolation and characterization of special compounds possessed with unique chemical and antibacterial properties ushered in a new era for antibiotics.

At about the same time as Hotchkiss and Dubos announced the isolation of two distinct and active peptides, called gramicidin and tyrocidine, from *Bacillus brevis,* a re-evaluation of the chemotherapeutic possibilities of Fleming's penicillin was published by Chain, Florey, et al. (1940) in England. During this same period, the investigations of actinomycetes carried on by Waksman and colleagues (1942) led to the discovery and isolation of streptothricin. Later streptomycin was prepared, and this compound proved to be a very important therapeutic drug. The ideology and methodology developed by these independent groups of workers had a tremendous impact on the quiescent area of antibiotics with the result that a new discipline was created to go hand in hand with Paul Ehrlich's school of chemotherapeutics which had already contributed salvarsan and sulfonamides. When once the way had been pointed out, numerous laboratory groups set to work in earnest, and as a result a very large list of antibiotic compounds has been discovered in the decade 1940-1950.

### TECHNIQUES OF THE QUEST

As an aid in the search for organisms which produce antibiotic substances, simple techniques have been developed which are applicable to the survey of large numbers of cultures. Small samples of soil, compost, or other materials are collected from likely places. A portion of the sample is suspended in water and shaken for the purpose of dispersing cells or spores of the microorganisms present. Then a small amount of the liquid containing various kinds of microorganisms is spread over the surface of nutrient agar in glass dishes. After being allowed to incubate for several days, these dishes are usually covered with growths of many kinds of organisms. Sometimes where the colonies of these are crowded, obvious antagonisms become evident from the interference zones which form around active groups of organisms. The desired kinds of fungi or bacteria are carefully transplanted one at a time so as to obtain pure cultures, i.e., one kind of organism growing by itself in a suitable medium. These cultures are tested in simple ways for their ability to prevent growth of certain selected strains of microbes.

One common method is the streak plate technique, in which the potential producer of an antibiotic substance is first grown on a portion of an agar plate, and then appropriate test organisms are seeded into the plate near the potential donor organism. After sufficient time has been allowed for growth of the indicators, the plate is inspected for zones of growth inhibition near the points of contact between the potential donor and receiver. Several test strains may be streaked on the same agar plate at right angles to the line of growth made by the first organism.

*Paul R. Burkholder*

Promising antibiotic cultures are usually grown in agitated nutrient broth for several days and then the beers are assayed against pathogenic organisms or other indicator strains. One very convenient method of making this assay is by placing on an agar plate, seeded with test bacteria, sterile filter-paper pads impregnated with the antibiotic solution. Glass cylinders may also be used, but the paper pads are more convenient. Zones of inhibition can be used as an indication of the potency of substances active against the test organisms. Broth dilution tests are sometimes made in order to find out what dilutions of a substance will inhibit the growth of test bacteria in a suitable liquid medium. In the plate test or broth assay, relative growth inhibition by a sample can be compared with that given by purified or standardized substances. Each laboratory has its own special methods for surveying organisms and developing suitable media for efficient production of antibiotics. For determining the activity of larger organisms, such as fleshy fungi, lichens and flowering plants, buffered water extracts of the materials are prepared and then applied to test organisms in petri plates or in broth tubes, just as in case of using the fermented beers of microorganisms.

With perseverance it is relatively easy to find numerous cultures of soil organisms which show microbial antagonism. The important question which now confronts the investigator is: which of his many cultures produce new, and interesting, and valuable antibiotic substances? He may employ several means of discovering whether some well-known substance is being formed by a freshly isolated microorganism. In the first place it is possible to study the colonial and micromorphology and physiology of the organism and thus attempt to compare it with other known antibiotic species or strains. Also, advantage can be taken of the fact that different strains of microorganisms vary greatly in their sensitivity to any particular antibiotic substance. The distinct differences observed in the susceptibility of various kinds of organisms to any given antibiotic allows the construction of a chart known as an antibiotic spectrum. The pattern of this spectrum, consisting of a list of microbes, some of which are resistant and others susceptible to the substance, sometimes throws considerable light upon the identity of any new compound being investigated, or the strain of organism being studied. By cross-streaking on an agar plate antibiotic-producing organisms, which are resistant to the known substances which they make, together with the new organism being studied, it is sometimes possible to derive valuable data concerning the nature of the substance formed by the new culture. Furthermore, it is possible in many instances to develop antibiotic-resistant strains out of susceptible cultures by their continued exposure to suitable concentrations of a drug. Such drug-resistant strains can serve as precise indicators to be used in identification of unknowns. Thus, if a streptomycin-resistant strain of bacteria is found to be susceptible to products of a new isolate obtained from soil, then it can be concluded that among these products is a substance different from streptomycin.

When the biological data indicate that a substance has interesting and perhaps unique properties, it is desirable to study some of the chemical and physical characteristics. By differential solubility in solvents and by precipitation techniques, it may be feasible to concentrate and purify the active agent. By the use of paper chromatography we have been investigating the mobility of known antibiotics, and by obtaining data on the relative fronts of known and un-

unidentified substances it is possible oftentimes to determine whether the activity of an unknown is ascribable to a well-known compound or whether it is something different.

## ANTIBIOTICS AND CHEMOTHERAPY

The therapeutic value of the known antibiotic substances varies greatly because of differences in sensitivity of disease-producing microbes to any given antibiotic material and because of tremendous differences in the toxicity of various compounds when administered to animals and man. Although more than one hundred and fifty antibiotics have been described so far, only a few, such as penicillin, streptomycin, bacitracin, chloromycetin, tyrothricin, aureomycin, and terramycin, have thus far been found suitable for extensive use in medicine. What are the requirements which have to be met so that an antibiotic may become a valuable chemotherapeutic? Some of these may be discussed here briefly as they bear upon the selection of substances greatly desired for urgent human needs. ·

The special goal of chemotherapy is the eradication of pathogenic forms of life with a minimum of effect upon the tissues and metabolic processes of the host. Effective chemotherapeutics do not act primarily on the host, but rather combine chemically with the parasite and act like monkey wrenches in the metabolic machinery of the pathogenic organism. The criterion of usefulness of a drug was summarized in Paul Ehrlich's concept of chemotherapeutic ratio which refers to the ratio of the dose which just produces toxic effects in the host to that which is required to get rid of the parasite. In present-day parlance the chemotherapeutic index = maximum tolerated dose/minimum effective dose.

The main points of importance in the development of agents useful in clinical practice are the following: (1) the discovery by isolation or synthesis of compounds which inhibit the parasite at some reasonable concentration *in vitro,* (2) selection of drugs which yield a satisfactory therapeutic ratio, (3) studies on practical means of administration so as to bring the drug into chemical union with the parasite, (4) application of the agent in controlled clinical studies to evaluate the performance of the drug as a practical therapeutic agent. The goal is to establish and maintain in the patient effective drug levels exceeding the *in vitro* predetermined threshold level of inhibition for the pathogen without causing undue harm to the patient. It is always hoped that organisms initially sensitive to an antibiotic will not readily develop resistance to its action. An ideal chemotherapeutic substance should be administered by the oral route, then be slowly and completely absorbed, bound preferentially to the proteins of the pathogen rather than those of the host, selectively active against important or unique vital steps in the metabolism of the disease-producing organisms, leaving the machinery of the host tissues unharmed, not appreciably inactivated by the microbial or body enzymes, and finally slowly excreted in the urine. Though the ideal drug has never been found, still the science of medicine has progressed a long way toward the goal. As an example, penicillin constitutes a pharmacologic curiosity because of its almost completely innocuous character coupled with a very great activity against certain kinds of pathogenic bacteria. Chloromycetin is active against gram-negative bacteria and Rickettsiae, and at effective dosage levels shows no harmful side reactions in man. Unfortunately, many substances can never measure up to the rigorous standards demanded in practical therapy. Actinomycin, for example, is very active against many microorganisms, but its great toxicity precludes any application in internal medicine. So it is with a large number of toxic antibiotics.

Antibiotics show great variation in their biological activity and their physical and chemical characteristics depending upon the source, whether from a species of actinomycete, a bacterium, some kind of mold or a green plant. Certain organisms produce more than one kind of antibiotic substance in the metabolic transformations which they bring about in suitable solutions of minerals and organic nutrients. Thus, *Bacillus brevis* produces gramicidin and tyrocidin. *Penicillium* molds produce several different types of penicillin, and in addition, also notatin. Another mold, *Aspergillus fumigatus,* forms spinulosin, fumigatin, fumigacin, and gliotoxin. Some antibiotics are produced by more than just one kind of microorganism. Thus, penicillin is made by many strains of *Penicillium* and *Aspergillus,* and actinomycin and streptomycin are produced by different kinds of actinomycetes belonging to the genus *Streptomyces.*

All too often without adequate knowledge concerning the chemistry of the two compounds being studied, special names have been assigned to antibiotic substances occurring in fermented broths or in crude preparations derived from different microorganisms. Considerable confusion may develop by creating, for one and the same antibiotic substance, different names assigned according to the nomenclature of the organisms producing the observed antimicrobial activity. Thus, the term clavacin was given to a certain antibiotic observed in the culture broth of *Aspergillus clavatus.* The same active principle isolated from *Penicillium claviforme* was called claviformin; but when it came from *P. patulum,* the substance was known as patulin; and when derived from *P. expansum* it was called expansine. In some instances quite similar but not identical antibiotics are produced by organisms widely separated in taxonomy, e.g., the seven carbon-ring compounds thujaplicin made by the tree, *Thuja plicata,* and puberulic acid formed by the mold, *Penicillium puberulum.* Although the source and antibiotic activity against various microorganisms provide valuable information, the proper identification of antibiotics rests finally upon the elucidation of the physical and chemical properties of the compounds.

Many diverse structural forms are represented among the numerous kinds of molecules which show antibiotic activity. Some of the simpler compounds are made of the elements C, H, and O as, for example, in the case of kojic acid ($C_6H_6O_4$) or spinulosin ($C_8H_8O_5$). Other more complicated structures may contain nitrogen as in streptomycin ($C_{12}H_{37}O_{12}N_7$), and also sulfur, as in gliotoxin ($C_{13}H_{14}N_2O_4S_2$) and the penicillins ($C_9H_{11}O_4SN_2$–R). Other types of antibiotics may contain chlorine, as in ustin ($C_{19}H_{15}O_5Cl_3$), chloromycetin ($C_{11}H_{12}O_5N_2Cl_2$) and aureomycin. A group of bacterial compounds, iodinin, pyocyanin, hemipyocyanin and chlororaphin, contain the heterocyclic phenazine nucleus. Another group of substances have in common the presence of an unsaturated lactone ring, as for example, clavacin, gladiolic acid, dicumarol and penicillic acid. Quinones constitute an important type of antibiotic, represented by citrinin, fumagatin, and spinulosin. Some quinones were isolated from fungi long before their antibiotic properties were suspected. In the class of polypeptides are such substances as gramicidin and subtilin, and the still more complex proteins are represented by the colicins and actinomycetin.

Antibiotics differ from each other markedly with regard to the effect of the medium upon their antimicrobial activities. Some materials, such as blood, proteins, etc., may diminish the activity and cause great reduction in the potency of the compound when tested *in vivo* as compared with assays against organisms *in vitro*. Some kinds of bacteria elaborate enzymes which destroy antibiotics. Penicillinase, an enzyme made by such common bacteria as *Escherichia coli* and many others also, readily inactivates penicillin, whereas streptomycin is usually highly resistant to the enzymatic action of microbes.

## THE FUTURE OF ANTIBIOTICS

One may stop to consider why the quest for new antibiotic compounds proceeds at an ever-increasing pace in numerous university and industrial laboratories around the world. The story of antibiotics began with those who labored for the love of academic learning, and still today such research is not without value for an understanding of the ways of life. Knowledge concerning the machinery of living cells and the principles of co-operation and conflict which have developed among the lower organisms, still evolving along with men on the earth, may help us to appreciate whence we have come and where we may be going. Studies on the properties of growth-promoting and growth-inhibiting substances and research on the action of antimetabolites, the synthetic analogs of vitamins and various other components of cellular architecture, all truly converge upon the fundamental goals of experimental biology. By investigating specific modes of antibiotic action, one may be led to discover important mechanisms of cellular activity. Preliminary glimpses into the chemistry of natural antibiotic compounds will doubtless open new vistas to be explored by the synthetic chemists who believe in the possibilities of making the right kind of molecules for a rational chemotherapy.

Even though wonderful drugs are now available, more and different kinds are needed for use against the new disease-producing microbes, which continue to develop resistance to the drugs once used effectively against their progenitors. Bacteria in some instances become adapted to withstand relatively high concentrations of a drug, even several thousand times the levels which formerly were inhibitory. The varied phenomena of drug adaptation are of great interest to academic biologists studying genetics and biochemistry, as well as to the clinician who is concerned with the universal struggle against disease. The adaptation of pathogenic microbes to antibiotics during treatment of a disease can be explained on the basis of spontaneous mutation from drug sensitivity to drug tolerance, and subsequent selection of the resistant offspring which are favored through elimination of associated competing drug-susceptible microorganisms in the mixed microbial population. It is fortunate that such adaptations are usually quite specific. Bacteria which have become resistant to streptomycin still may retain the susceptibility to penicillin which they possessed initially. Refractory medical cases need not involve lack of co-operation on the part of the patient, but may sometimes be explained by the evolution of drug-tolerant microbes causing the diseased condition. A knowledge of the drug tolerance of pathogenic bacteria is needed before adequate dosages can be formulated. Combined medication with mixtures of drugs and adjuvants appears to provide insurance against mutant microbes and a means of shortening the duration of required medical treatment. The preparation of slightly modified drug derivatives, resembling the general pattern of a natural antibiotic, may also prove to be helpful in overcoming drug-fast organisms.

The pattern of growth in research and publication of scientific papers in the whole field of antibiotics during the past fifty years suggests that the subject is well under way toward its peak of development. How many more good antibiotics remain to be developed for chemotherapy no one really knows. We can be certain, however, that the necessity of finding new cures for man's physical ills will be before us for a long while. The few antibiotics and other antimicrobial drugs now available to the medical profession are useful in the treatment of coccal infections, intestinal disorders, skin diseases, and even severe Rickettsial infections. But what about the common cold, polio, tuberculosis, and cancer? The need for dependable means of chemotherapy against these and many other scourges of mankind is very great. One can only hope that effective checks may be found to stop the peculiar growth and multiplication of small viruses, the tubercle bacilli, and the dreaded malignant cells which all too frequently arise in the human body. The quest for antibiotics requires arduous and painstaking work, but the stakes for human health are high. Many trained workers with vision and self-discipline are needed to carry on. The rewards to those who succeed in finding the goal of their explorations are measured in recognition of high services to their fellow men.

## REFERENCES

Baron, A. L. (1950), *Handbook of Antibiotics.* New York: Reinhold.

Florey, H. W. et al. (1949), *Antibiotics,* 2 Vols. London: Oxford University Press.

Irving, G. W. and H. T. Herrick (1949), *Antibiotics.* New York: Chemical Publishing Co.

Pratt, R. and J. Dufrenoy (1949), *Antibiotics.* Philadelphia: Lippincott Co.

# STRESS, EMOTIONS AND
# BODILY DISEASE

## By Harold G. Wolff, M.D.

OUR LANGUAGE bears witness to the fact that men have long known that certain life experiences, feelings, and bodily changes are connected. Let me remind you by quoting a few phrases picked out of everyday experience that indicate this general knowledge:

He was red in the face; he was hot under the collar; he was blushing; he was pale with rage; he was in the pink of condition; it brought tears to his eyes; his eyes popped out of his head; his tongue clove to the roof of his mouth; his mouth was filled with cotton wool; it took one's breath away; he breathed heavily with passion; he got into a cold sweat; cold hands, warm heart; cold feet; dripping with suspense; it was a nauseating experience; it makes me sick; it turns my stomach; he had a lump in his throat; he got a weight off his chest; he's a pain in the neck; he's a gripe; he trembled with fear; he shook with rage; he has the jitters; he's a stiff-necked fellow; he's weak with laughter; keep a stiff upper lip; and, faint heart ne'er won fair lady.

Industry has not been blind to this problem, if I may call the moving picture an industry. A thousand people sweat approximately 100 lbs. of moisture in one hour under ordinary conditions, but under the emotionally charged conditions of a thrilling motion picture, the moisture output rises to 150 lbs.

There are two standard works, not textbooks of anatomy, that bear further witness to this fact. *Bartlett's Familiar Quotations* has in its index nine columns of phrases including the heart. There are few other words in the language—such as "life," "love," and "man"—that have more references. *Roget's Thesaurus* has the word "heart" in the index more often than any other single word. Indeed, the word "heart" has become a symbol of the human spirit: "hard-hearted," "warm-hearted," "cold-hearted," "steel-hearted," etc. Now obviously I'm dealing in truisms. You well know what I say to be true—that we continually use words that indicate our knowledge that the body participates with our feelings and in reaction to experiences. However, what I would like to discuss with you this evening is: How pertinent are these changes to health? How much do they become the problem of the man who is concerned about his very life? In other words, when do these changes begin to disturb our effectiveness and sometimes to jeopardize our lives?

Now I propose to present to you the data from which some of our inferences are drawn. Some of the time, these will not be very tidy-looking facts, but I ask you to be tolerant and to realize that we are dealing with man, and man is made up not only of aspirations but of bowels as well.

SKIN

I will describe some observations relevant to the subject of this evening's discussion as it concerns the skin. Dr. David Graham performed the following experiment in which the capillary tone was tested in a subject's two arms for the ability of those vessels to hold the bloody contents within their walls. The left arm was then struck, quite forcefully, and immediately there appeared a red area which began to swell, a wale or a welt appeared, and the deterioration of the capillary tone was charted. But the right arm behaved in the same way even though it was not actually struck. The left arm gradually returned to its former state; the right arm reached that state a little sooner. In a little while, we repeated the experiment, except that now, instead of bringing the ferrule down onto the forearm, we brought it just short of the arm. It was a sham blow (Fig. 1). The left arm was seen to behave just as it did before even though no injury was inflicted. The right arm seemed to be a little wiser. It did not respond as before. Then gradually the left returned to its former state. In a little while we again repeated the whole procedure except that this time we told our subject what was going to happen, and after the sham blow nothing in the way of a body change took place. In other words, the individual, through his skin, was reacting to a blow by putting into his tissues a certain amount of fluid, perhaps representing a reaction to tissue injury on the one hand, and perhaps on the other, to protect him from further injury.

Now let us make a shift. A man came to us because of a complaint of hives. Again we made a record of the ability of his capillaries to hold onto their contents. This time instead of striking him with a ferrule, we discussed a situation involving his family which made him feel in many ways as though he were being hit. "Just thinking about things they did to me," was his answer when asked about his thoughts and feelings (Fig. 2). At the same time his arm behaved as though he were actually struck, and he developed welts or

Stress, Emotions and Bodily Disease

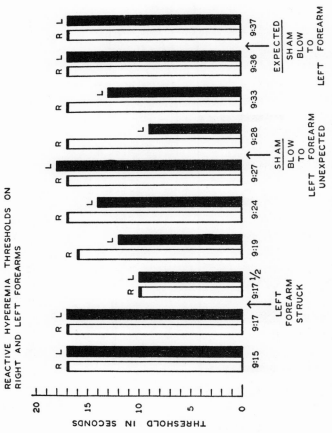

FIG. 1.—Changes in the reactive hyperemia threshold of both forearms of a healthy man in response to real and feigned blows to the left forearm.

97

*Harold G. Wolff*

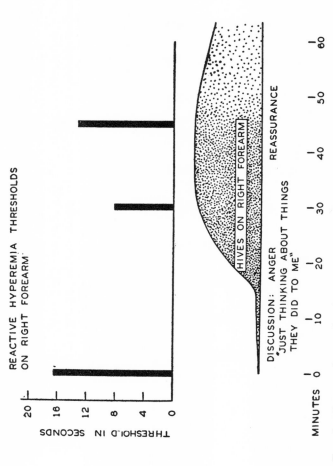

Fig. 2.—Lowered reactive hyperemia threshold while urticaria was developing, with return toward normal as lesions ceased to appear.

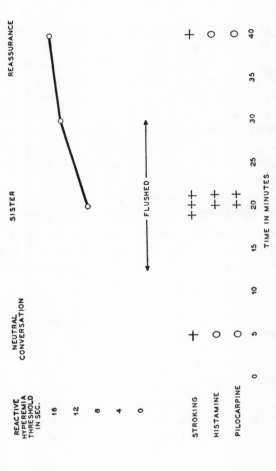

Fig. 3.—Simultaneous changes in the response of the skin to histamine, to pilocarpine, and to stroking during a stressful interview with a woman patient. (Histamine acid phosphate 0.001 per cent, and pilocarpine hydrochloride 1 per cent at only 10 microamperes for two minutes over 1 square centimeter.) There was no response to physiological saline applied in the same way before, during, and after the period of stress.

wales which we call, in his case, hives. In a little while, they disappeared. Notice, then, that the body pattern which serves to protect was used in a way in which it was of no special value.

Let us take this argument one step further. This time we first tested an individual's skin as regards its ability to react to stroking, to a chemical poison named histamine and to another one named pilocarpine. Note that his skin was insensitive to all of these (Fig. 3). We then exposed him to a troublesome discussion by introducing a topic which made him feel as though he were taking a beating and could do nothing about it. At the height of his reaction we saw the very same noxious stimuli, that before produced practically no effect, produce a great effect. In other words, he became vulnerable to a great many assaults at this time, not only to the effects which one might suppose would come from the discussion about his family troubles, but also to the other noxious influences. He was at that moment in a weakened or exposed state. In a little while, with reassurance, he returned to his original condition.

Stenographic records of what a subject says during such bodily changes were made by Dr. Graham and Dr. Grace. Here's what one hears during a conversation in which an individual is developing hives: "They did a lot of things to me and I couldn't do anything about it. I was getting pushed around. I had to sit and take it. I was taking a beating. They were cracking a whip over me. My mother is constantly hammering on me. He knocked me down and walked all over me." In other words, while his body is acting as though it were taking a beating, he feels as though he were being exposed to such assault. This, then, is the pattern that we are going to consider again and again. We find the organism dealing with an assault in a given way, and using that pattern again and again, sometimes in re-action to noxious interpersonal relations, where it can serve no useful or appropriate end.

Let us turn now to the stomach. Let us assume that we are measuring the blood flow in the first part of the small intestine or the last part of the stomach. The following is what occurred when we presented a person with a plate containing food: the food happened to interest him, and immediately the blood flow in the lining of his stomach in-creased. As the food was removed, the blood flow gradually returned to its original level. We took a record of what the stomach was doing mechanically and found that it was churning and contracting. We took a record of the secre-tions that have to do with digestion, and found that they too were increased in amount. In other words, this stomach was preparing for the act of digestion even though the in-dividual was only looking at food. Then we took a step further and again presented a plate of food, but this plate of food had no meaning to the individual. His appetite was not stimulated and there was no change in the conduct of the stomach. It did not prepare to digest.

Next, the food was removed from view, and instead of introducing something he could see, or smell, we intro-duced a few words. We considered with him some article of food that actually stimulated his appetite; immediately his stomach prepared to go into digestive activity. We were operating on a truly symbolic level, dealing with words that had to do with food rather than with food itself. Let us advance another step. We introduced a topic which was extremely noxious to this individual, a patient in the hos-pital. He was exceedingly angry because his partner, during his hospital stay, had exploited the patient's absence from his business to carry on some shady business deals and to bring disrepute upon his name. And as he discussed his partner's bad behavior, his duodenum and stomach acted as though they were preparing to digest. During this exhibition of anger, his upper gastrointestinal tract acted as though it were about to digest a meal.

This type of experimentation was greatly facilitated by the appearance in our laboratory of a man named Tom, now about sixty-five, who at the age of nine experienced a serious accident. He came home from school one day, thirsty and warm, and mistakenly drank some scalding hot clam chowder which occluded his gullet so that thereafter no food could enter his stomach. At that time, it was necessary, in order to keep him alive, to make a hole on the anterior portion of his abdomen, and through this hole he has since fed himself twice a day for half a century or more. This man has taken his place in life as citizen, father, a good worker, and a solid person. He is shy, taciturn, with strong feelings about "respectability" and his capacity to take his place in the community.

He has joined our laboratory group and daily comes into the laboratory where we measure the redness of his gastric mucosa or stomach lining, which indicates the amount of blood flow. The redder, the more blood flow; the paler, the less blood flow. We also ascertain the secretion of gastric juices and the churning activity. At the same time we take note of what is going on in his life: his fears, his hopes, his wishes, his frustrations, his satisfactions.

On one particular occasion, when Tom was resting on the laboratory table as was customary, one of my colleagues entered the room and said that a certain important protocol was missing. Tom was responsible for this protocol and realized that he was guilty of a major defection. He grew pale in face and gradually grew pale in his stomach as his terror increased. My colleague opened and closed drawers, muttering imprecations. He finally found the protocol, slammed the door and left. At this moment, our subject said, "I was scared that I had lost my job." This statement has to be seen in symbolic terms. The man was afraid that he had lost his position not only as our fellow worker, but as a human being who had been entrusted with responsibility. His stomach was pale, hypoactive, nondigestive, nonfunctioning. This stomach was "out of condition." It was associated with sensations of distension. When his stomach behaved in this way, digestion was slowed. He complained of flatulence, food remained in the stomach a long time, he experienced gaseous eructations, he often felt nauseated and sometimes vomited. Thus, you see an example of a hypofunctioning organ, an organ not preparing to digest under circumstances of stress.

In contrast with this, the following observation was made on our same subject, when, again resting on the table, he was confronted by the fact that a job of dusting and cleaning an apartment which he had undertaken for one of my colleagues was being improperly done. Tom, being an indifferent housekeeper, was not as meticulous about his dusting as one might have wished. So my colleague dispensed with his services under these circumstances of observation. As he was being told about his inadequacy, he got red in the face, red in the stomach, his acid increased in amount, his stomach began to churn, and, when told that he was "fired," it became exceedingly red. My colleague then left, having said what he had in mind to say to Tom, whereupon Tom spoke quite differently, muttering,

*Harold G. Wolff*

"I'd like to wring his neck." This was an expression of anger; he felt abused and "put upon."

These changes last not only minutes, but may last weeks. The acid secretion before, during a period of crisis and afterwards, and the color before, during the period of crisis and afterwards, are described in the following: Receiving a small salary, Tom was obliged to accept the kindness of a benefactor who meddled in his personal life. This was exceedingly irksome to Tom; his independence was threatened and he repeatedly made efforts to throw off his benefactor, but he could not. It was particularly irksome during a certain two-week period, at which time he exhibited a high acid secretion and a deep red color. It was possible with a slight raise in salary to rid himself of his benefactor, upon which his stomach returned to its former state.

A moving picture taken of Tom's stomach has taught us much. Food enters the bottom of his stomach through a hole, surrounded by a piece of the stomach extruded on the outside of the body. The color of his stomach as represented on the anterior abdominal wall is pink when there is an average amount of secretion. It gets very red, however, and very readily bleeds, so that even its own contractions, or touching it, or taking food on its surface causes damage. There is a dark red appearance, the ready bleeding which I mentioned, the increase in the amount of secretion, and the general swollen appearance of this mucosa when he now is threatened and angry at what he considers an unjust accusation. There are a myriad of small red spots, little hemorrhages that occurred during this period when it was so engorged. It becomes boggy and wet and swollen as a result of that long period of engorgement. The spots in this case lasted about seventy-two hours, after

*104*

which the mucous membrane appeared as it did originally. Those red spots may become quite important since some of them may be converted into ulcers. Also, one can see how one of these little tiny hemorrhages begins to be converted to an ulcer by allowing the digestive juices of the stomach to act upon it. Thus we have a cycle: from a dissatisfaction, a frustration, a resentment maintained, to a hole in the gastric mucosa.

Another man who presented a stoma, such as did our

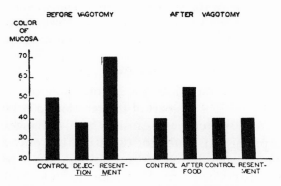

FIG. 4.—Variations in color of the gastric mucosa under a variety of circumstances before and after vagotomy.

subject Tom, gave us short-lived opportunities for examination because of his death. This man, to begin with, had mucosa of pink color. If we discussed with him a certain doctor who he believed had failed to do his duty by properly diagnosing his illness, he became exceedingly angry. His face was red, he sputtered, he became profane, he thumped the table, and his stomach mucosa became very dark red. It became necessary as part of his treatment to cut a certain nerve, known as the vagus nerve. After surgery, discussion of this same doctor, which was associated with every outward show of anger as exhibited before, was coupled with no such change in his stomach (Fig. 4). In other words, it is as though this man had his hand cut off; he could still feel angry, but he couldn't thump the table. In this last example, I present a picture of a man bombarded by life and having a variety of reactions to experience which, in terms of his past, are converted into certain patterns of action. They include, in this case, the sending of impulses down the vagus nerve which convert the mucous membrane of the stomach from a healthy state to one showing a hole, and possibly leading to the circumstances requiring surgery and perhaps other heroic measures.

### ATTITUDES

Let me draw certain inferences from these observations. First of all, emotions are part of the reaction to stress. They should not be spoken of as causing bodily changes. What one feels privately is truly not causative, but only another manifestation of an individual's reaction to his experience. In other words, when something happens to an individual, he develops an attitude which might be thought of as having two parts. First, what meaning has this experience for me? Am I threatened by it? Is it safe? Do I enjoy it? Must I fear it? What is its meaning to me? And secondly, what do I do about it? This may be going on consciously or, for the most part, unconsciously.

When an individual decides to get rid of something because it is disgusting or unattractive, as when he's vomiting, he expresses certain characteristic attitudes. Let me read you some of his statements as recorded by my colleagues Dr. Graham and Dr. Grace. A vomiting person expresses himself this way: "I wish it hadn't happened. I didn't want this. Something had happened which I wished hadn't happened. Why did it have to happen? I wish things were the way they were before. I wish I hadn't gotten into this. I wish I hadn't listened to him." It is as though the individual were trying to get out of him what he inadvertently admitted.

Must the mutual processes involved be unconscious? What is the role of the conscious? Much has been said concerning the conscious versus the unconscious. But far more relevant at the moment, it would seem to me, in our considerations of these matters, would be an appraisal of "What is the meaning of a situation for the individual?" Very often, meaningful, important matters are so dreadful, so overwhelming that they are dismissed from consciousness and therefore disappear from awareness of the individual. If it be conscious, then at least it has a chance of being dealt with. If it is unconscious, it may remain in the category where it is less accessible and the individual suffers its effects for long periods. But I repeat: the important matter for our consideration is, "What is the meaning of an experience, or a stimulus, or a threat, or a statement?" And then, "What do I do about it?"

### BOWEL

Now having had some contact with the human insides, let us go to the other end of the gastrointestinal tract, the large bowel, and see what general information, what general principles can be derived. We have had four individuals who have had pieces of their large bowel on the outside of the body, so placed surgically for various and very good reasons. These exposures gave us an opportunity to study the connection of the bowel with life experiences. (Let me add, parenthetically, that these people are really saints; they have dedicated their damaged bodies to the pursuit of truth, as we understood it, and have selflessly co-operated in giving us what we asked them.)

Let us begin with this simple experiment. A man had a thumb screw arrangement put on his head. The man knew that he was going to be hurt. Squeezing his head with the thumb screws caused his bowel to get red and to contract. He felt angry and anxious, but placidly accepted the assault. A second man, despite the fact that he wished to participate and knew what we were going to do, had, in reaction to exactly the same stimulus, under the same circumstances, in the same room on the same day, precisely the opposite reaction. His bowel got pale, and contractile activity stopped. A general principle is exemplified: here were two people exposed to the same assault, yet presenting opposite reactions. The assault had a different "meaning" for one than it did for the other. The fact of individuality becomes immediately apparent.

A person's bowel when he is in a state of relative tranquility is pink in color. During a period of dejection or sadness, it becomes pale and relaxed. During a period of anger, it is dark red and contracted, and becomes hypermotile when a balloon is inserted within the lumen. The bowel, about twenty minutes after eating, becomes red and hypermotile during a period of tranquillity. This is the so-called gastrocolic reflex and is the basis of the urge to defecate after meals. The same individual under ostensibly the same circumstances may react to lunch not at all as regards any change in color or blood supply to his mucosa, or the contractile state of his guts when he is dejected because of an incident in relation to a neighbor just a few hours before.

### THE SIGNIFICANCE OF THE TOPIC

Now I would emphasize that when in an interview we touch upon a topic that sets off a reaction, it does not mean that this is a key situation in the individual's life and that if this particular difficulty could be solved, all difficulties would disappear. But it means that the topic under discussion is representative of many situations which would be looked upon as threats in the same way, and reacted to in a similar way. For example, we discussed with a very sensitive man something about his sister-in-law. This man's bowel trouble, known as ulcerative colitis, or ulceration of the bowel, began shortly after the death of his mother. He was the eldest son, sensitive, passive, excessively dependent on her words and acts of affection. He was devastated by the loss caused by her death. He became the head of the family, a position he assumed with vigor, but without effectiveness. His younger brother married and brought into the home a woman who threatened our patient's security and challenged his position as head of the family. Merely discussing this woman and her attitudes and behavior in the family setting caused his bowel to become contracted and dark red. His sister-in-law had become a threatening symbol, and this man reacted to other threats to his security in the same manner. The bowel acted as though it were trying in a simple manner to get rid of this situation which obviously was not to be got rid of so simply.

Another individual's reactions to his troubles may be described. He was a sailor who believed that because of his religious affiliations he was not given a "good berth" on ships. Discussion of this topic caused his feelings to be aroused, anger expressed, and his bowels to contract and become red. He was easily diverted, however, and in a few minutes the bowel was paler and relaxed. Again, in a few minutes, he felt very much threatened and challenged by his misinterpretation of questions which he took to indicate that we doubted his integrity. Again the bowel became dark red and contracted.

Constipation and diarrhea are opposites in their functional significance. Diarrhea, designed to help the organism get rid of some noxious agent it had inadvertently admitted by mouth or otherwise, is associated with increased redness and heightened motility of the bowel, so that as quickly as possible the noxious agent may be emitted. Constipation, on the other hand, the opposite state, is associated with a large, relaxed, pale bowel showing ineffective contractions, with retention of the ingested substances for longer than the usual periods, perhaps with contraction of the skeletal muscles around the outlet further to impede the disposition of the bowel contents. It constitutes a good-sized medical problem in our time and often alternates with diarrhea. I will describe in a moment some of the things which patients with constipation feel, what their attitudes toward life can be said to be at that time. But in the individual with a hypermotile gut, red, overcontracted, the mucous membrane becomes very fragile. When a person is relaxed and tranquil, a negative pressure of about 100 or more mm. of mercury is easily withstood for six minutes, or, even 200 mm., without bleeding. But when a person is insecure and angry and his bowel is in an overactive, inflamed state, it takes very little, say 60 mm. of mercury pressure for one and a half minutes, or even the individual's own contractions, to cause the tissue to tear and bleed. Under these circumstances, when bleeding so readily occurs, many small erosions and ulcers appear on the gut. In other words, this exposed portion of mucous membrane goes to pieces under circumstances that can have little to do with the colonic content of the feces. These areas are damaged by erosion or ulceration. They are often the sites of serious hemorrhage and occasionally cause death.

Now, what is the opposite side of the coin? A patient bleeding profusely from the bowels, with fever and considerable weight loss, makes contact with another human being who helps alter his attitude toward life, re-establish his self-esteem, re-establish his faith and trust in himself and others. His temperature becomes normal, he gains in weight, and the bloody diarrhea, which is an inappropriate expression of the desire to get rid of something, stops.

Thus, a stressful life circumstance or a symbol thereof evokes certain protective reactions—in a particular instance, the desire to get rid of something by pushing it out of the gut. Vomiting at one end of the gut has riddance as its goal; diarrhea at the other, has a similar function. The individual feels angry, resentful, hostile, as well as anxious and apprehensive, though passive. At the same time, not closely related but concurrently manifesting itself, is altered function of the colon, with increased contractility, increased blood flow, engorgement, alteration of secretion, with bleeding, tearing of the gut, erosions, ulcerations, hemorrhages and perhaps secondary infection.

What does such a person feel? What attitude does he express at the time that this pattern is being fulfilled? The individual with diarrhea or ulcerative colitis says: "I wanted to be done with it." "I want this to be finished." "I want it to be all over." "If I can only get rid of it." I remind you that often men facing a firing line have diarrhea. In contrast, the individual with constipation, grimly determined to carry on, even though faced with a problem he cannot solve, says the following: "This is a lousy job, but it is the best I can get. I will have to keep on with this, but I know I'm not going to like it. It will never be any better, but I will keep on with what I have. I don't want to do it, but I will go through with it. It's no good, but I won't quit. I don't get any fun out of it, but I keep on doing it."

### THE INTERPRETATION OF BODILY CHANGES

How are we to look at these bodily changes? Are they accidents? When a person is under stress, might anything happen? Is it fortuitous that one organ is used rather than another? This seems unlikely, because there is too much predictability about it. One individual under stress will get diarrhea again and again, another constipation, another vomiting, and still another a bleeding stomach. Is this a state only of general excitement so that with spread of excitation any sort of change may occur? Evidence to the contrary is that in the general excitement that occurs during battle, it is uncommon for a person to develop asthma, for example, or bleeding from a peptic ulcer. On the other hand, is some special isolated part of the nervous system involved? No. There is no evidence of any pure isolated response representing the activity of only one part of the nervous system. Thus, one cannot think of the reaction in terms of the function of any unique segment of the nervous system, or any special endocrine organ or gland.

How, then, should we think of it? To me, the most attractive notion is that the individual is using at such times of stress protective or adaptive patterns which have in their literal application a highly useful purpose: to meet a crisis, to maintain nutrition, or to help the individual adapt under such circumstances of duress. When dealing with a poison, it is good to vomit or have diarrhea.

When dealing with one's sister-in-law, it is of no use. In the latter instance, it is an inappropriate and excessively prolonged pattern of action, designed for a good end but used awkwardly and, because of that, used excessively, and thus perhaps damaging the individual or destroying the life which it was designed to protect.

I would not have you take the view that these patterns of a protective nature serve no purpose. For example, you all know—anyone who has wept, and all have wept—that a good display of tears will often make one feel better. Any pattern in action brings with it a degree of tranquillity. We feel a little better after running, jumping, crying out, weeping, vomiting, even though nothing has been solved. So there is something to be obtained, but the harmful feature is that the price is often high and, if we continue in the pattern too long, we may damage our tissues and get into further trouble. Therefore we stand accused of an uneconomic and inappropriate use of our equipment, and are punished accordingly.

### AIRWAYS

Now I'd like to take you into another department of the body, that having to do with the airways. I suppose by this time you are saying to yourself, "Well everybody doesn't get an ulcer of the stomach or trouble with the large intestine or hives. Why is it that we behave differently?" Let's postpone the question, but let me show you that we do act in different ways. Let us take as an example a person we examined as regards the color of nasal mucous membrane by simply looking into the nose. Day in and day out he went along in a rather steady way as contrasted with another individual who exhibited most violent disturbances. This latter individual's nasal mucous membranes were red one day and pale the next, red on one side and pale on the other.

What is the meaning of such a change? I suggest that you take this experiment into consideration. We sat our friend down before a bottle of smelling salts. He reacted in the same manner in which most individuals react. It is a familiar experience, and you all know what happens. The individual suddenly gasps, and the mucous membrane of

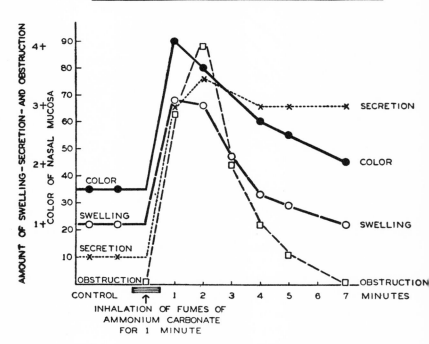

FIG. 5.—Hyperemia with swelling, hypersecretion, and obstruction of the nose following inhalation of noxious chemical agent, ammonium carbonate.

the nose gets very red and swollen (Fig. 5). Water pours out and hardly any air can get through. The individual may not be able to speak. His chest seems held in a vise, and the swelling in the upper airways could be seen if one were to look further down than the nose. It looks very much as though this human organism were attempting to neutralize, wash away, and shut out some very unattractive aspect

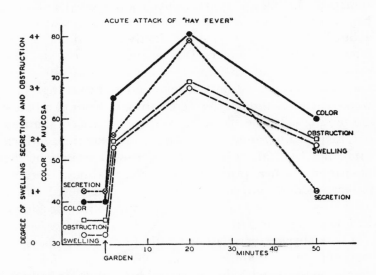

Fig. 6.—Hyperemia, hypersecretion, and obstruction in the nose during an abortive attack of hay fever.

of the environment. Well, the same thing happened when our sensitive friend went into the rose garden and was exposed to rose pollen. He developed, not hay fever, but what is similar to hay fever and his nose acted exactly the same way as it did when exposed to smelling salts (Fig. 6). He attempted seemingly to shut out, wash away, and neutralize this noxious agent to which he had been exposed.

Well, that's all very simple, and seems a proper use of the nose.

But consider a woman who came in with a long history of nose trouble. She'd had many operations. She was in for another. She couldn't get any air. Her nose seemed to be stopped up much of the time, especially at night, and, I might add, especially when her husband was in the room smoking. During an interview it was suggested that perhaps her troubles were in some way related to her attitudes about her husband. This she violently rejected and at the same time burst into tears. During the interview, the mucous membrane on the inside of her nose was quite red, and there was a good deal of secretion and swelling. This woman acted as though she were sitting in front of a bottle of smelling salts. She was acting as though she were shutting out, neutralizing, and washing away some experience which could not be dealt with in those terms. Throughout the discussion of her problems the woman's nose became pinker, redder, and more swollen, wet and closed off. A little while later, it was pale, boggy and solidly occluded, with nothing going through.

These changes may last not only minutes but days, as exhibited by an ambitious young physician who felt very much concerned with his career and his ambitions and was obliged to work in his hospital duties with a man some years his senior, but his junior in experience and wisdom. He very much resented working with this colleague, and constantly feared that his future would be jeopardized because of the inadequate performance of his associate. Their relations deteriorated rapidly. During a two-week period when his conflicts with this colleague were most severe, he had a very red mucous membrane, very much swollen, with a good deal of fluid pouring out, and hardly any air going in. During the period of his forced sojourn with this man, he developed headache which was called sinus headache, characterized by red eyes, tender, swollen cheeks and tender forehead. And when his mucous membranes were examined inside, they were exceedingly sensitive to touch, swollen, red and obviously inflamed. We observed that this man not only had this reaction but that during an interview, his mucous membranes began to swell and secretion poured out, and large quantities of pus cells appeared in the secretion. This is evidence of the kind of tissue change which experience with another man could bring about. It was possible to separate these individuals, and then our friend had a much paler mucous membrane, not so swollen, with practically no secretion and no obstruction.

In the following instance we have evidence of a summative effect, in which one kind of noxious stimulus is added to another. A patient was brought into a room containing pollen, constant in amount. He was very sensitive to the pollen, and as he rested in this room, his mucous membrane began to get red and swollen. Then, in addition to the pollen, we introduced a topic concerning his relations with his father. Immediately his symptoms were augmented and he could not breathe. He was reassured about his relations with his father, and, despite the fact that he remained in the room laden with pollen, the reassurances seemed able to restore his membrane to a state equivalent to that which existed before he entered the pollen-laden room. In this case, then, the more important noxious agent seemed to be the individual's relation to his father rather than the pollen, although both were operating.

An anatomical defect, present since birth, can begin to take on importance in middle life or later. For example, a deviated septum which has been there all one's life may become important when one's relations to one's colleagues get to be of such a nature as to call forth this protective reaction of shutting out, washing away, and neutralizing. A man in such a plight may need to have his septum removed to allow more air to get through.

This discussion would be incomplete if I were to leave out asthma, since we know that the asthmatic individual is closely akin to the one who has trouble with his nose, or may even be the same individual. We know by direct inspection of the mucous membranes that unpleasant topics cause the mucous membranes of the bronchi to become red and wet. During a series of observations we discussed topics calling forth such feelings as bitterness, regret and failure, and precipitated asthmatic attacks (Fig. 7).

You have often experienced, I dare say, a feeling of air hunger, and "butterflies in the stomach." One feels as though one were fluttering, under circumstances of tension. There may be a tight, unpleasant feeling of pressure in the middle of the chest, sometimes cramplike, taken for pains coming from the heart. Sometimes individuals are much disturbed by these sensations. Let me describe what is seen when an X-ray photograph of the diaphragm when an individual is relaxed and tranquil is superimposed upon an X-ray of the same individual when he is anxious and disturbed because of an experience with another human being. Comparison of the shadow of the diaphragm before he was upset, and the shadow after he has put a cramp, so to speak, in his sheet of muscle that connects the front of him with his back shows a state in which it would be difficult to take in more air. There is a kind of fluttering sensation which is associated with that, and there may be a cramplike sensation just underneath the heart giving rise to the symptoms of which we have just spoken.

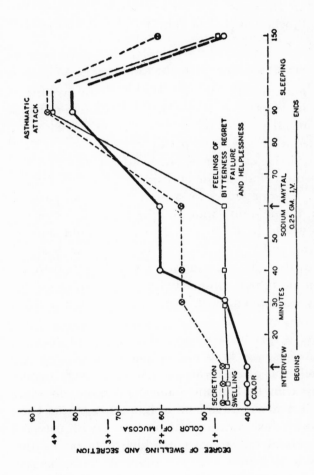

Fig. 7.—Experimentally induced hyperemia, swelling, hypersecretion, and obstruction in the nose associated with narrowing of the bronchial tubes during a discussion of topics provocative of feelings of remorse, guilt, and resentment.

*Harold G. Wolff*

The foregoing observations were made by my colleagues. Those on the nose were made by Dr. Holmes, those on the large bowel by Dr. Grace, and those on the stomach by Dr. Stewart Wolf, who has pursued kindred topics with me for many years.

## SPECIFICITY OF REACTIONS TO STRESS

Now let me epitomize what I have said. In evoking a protective or adaptive reaction, individuals don't necessarily call out all parts of the reaction pattern. That is to say, if one wished really to keep out, or wash away, or shut out an unattractive experience, one wouldn't stop with the nose. One would close off the entire airway system. But, as a matter of fact, one settles for a piece, or a small part, of the pattern. If one didn't want to take something into the stomach, it would be be supposed that one could start at the beginning and not swallow, or not chew, or close off the gullet, or that the large intestine would participate in the reaction of refusal. But actually, only pieces of the pattern may become engaged. This fragmentation is characteristic.

Also, there is specificity about stress. Any kind of stress doesn't evoke just any kind of reaction.

Let me tell you of observations made by a very distinguished physician in Holland named Jacob Groen who, during the bad years of Holland's occupation by the Germans, was able to examine a number of his Jewish patients who had ulcers of the stomach. He saw them before the Germans came and attended their medical needs; he saw them after they were put in concentration camps. For the most part, they were wealthy, "well-heeled," comfortable, successful merchants. They lived on the best streets and were well-clothed. They suffered a good deal with their stomachs.

When they got into concentration camps, obviously their lives were jeopardized. They never knew at the beginning of the day whether they would survive that day. There was endless quarreling, bickering, snarling, snapping, stealing; one national group hated the other national group. Certainly, life was as filled with stress as was possible for humans to endure; yet these individuals lost all manifestations of their peptic ulceration. And the ironic aspect of it is that many of them regained their peptic ulcers when they returned to Main Street. Now you cannot say that stress was lacking in the concentration camp, but that a specific type of stress which engendered the hole in the stomach in the first place was absent in the second.

I have cared for a group of patients with serious headaches who were missionaries in Japan. During the heyday of their effective missionary activity, they suffered considerably, even though esteemed and presumably satisfied, or at least effective, in their life effort. When these individuals were put into Japanese concentration camps, with the deprivations that were entailed, they lost their headaches, only to get them back when they were freed at the end of the war. At this time I can't go any further with this thesis except to point out that these instances indicate that stress has to have a specific meaning to the individual in order to produce the specific changes which I am calling to your attention.

In using these protective or adaptive patterns, individuals often enough pick out one, sometimes two patterns, and they may change. Thus, an individual may at one time have vascular headaches, and at another time have peptic ulcer; sometimes he may have them both at the same time.

*Harold G. Wolff*

Certain combinations are uncommon, such as ulcers of the large bowel and ulcers of the stomach. They seem to represent quite different ways of meeting danger.

I have thus given you evidence of tissue derangement as a part of an adjustment which was meant to protect the individual. I brought to you evidence about swelling, edema, reduction of blood supply to tissue, tenderness, inflammation, erosion, hemorrhage, ulceration, pus formation, changes in secretion, and lowering of the pain threshold.

OVER-ALL MOBILIZATION PATTERNS

I would next like to consider with you some over-all patterns. What I have given you so far are pieces of patterns, involving the mouth, or airways, or portals of entry, or the rectum, or anus, or portals of exit. Let us see what the organism can do by way of general mobilization for action. If a man runs upstairs or exercises vigorously, this is the kind of thing he does: he increases the amount of blood that his heart puts out, each stroke contains more blood than it did before, his heart rate is increased, his blood pressure goes up somewhat and he decreases the amount of resistance that is offered by the tissues of the body in accepting the blood that is brought to them.

Similarly, in an interview in which some important relationship to another human being is discussed, which causes him to be anxious and frightened, an individual acts just as though he were running upstairs, or preparing for battle, or preparing to run away. A patient came to us one February, in a tense, anxious, unhappy state, complaining of pounding heart and breathlessness. Climbing a certain number of steps caused this individual's already rapid, already much augmented stroke volume—that is to say, the amount of blood coming out of the heart with each contraction—to be further increased. The heart rate also was increased. As time went on, the patient's state gradually improved as his adjustment improved until, in December of the same year, precisely the same effort produced a minimal but effective response. At this time, he was a relatively tranquil, relaxed person doing easily what had to be done, whereas, before, this slight effort called forth a great energy output.

Let me describe a situation created by an interview with a man concerning his mother, whom he ostensibly loved but actually hated, never admitting this to himself and certainly to no one else. He presented a bland exterior during the interview, but at the same time his blood pressure rose and the resistance offered to the passage of blood by blood vessels of many of the organs mounted. His blood became much stickier and coagulated, or clotted more readily. When this man was interviewed concerning his relations with his mother, his blood pressure went up a great deal and, as a part of his generally increased resistance to the flow of blood, the amount of blood that went through the kidneys was much decreased. At the same time, with increased stickiness and clotting proclivity of the blood, he might further have damaged organs. This clotting device is designed presumably to help the animal stop bleeding should he be in mortal combat. But when it is used every time a person comes in contact with his mother, or some surrogate of his mother, you can see how he might appreciably damage his organs, notably his kidneys and perhaps his brain. Again, a device designed to protect and prolong the life of the individual is called into action so inappropriately as to threaten his very existence.

On the other hand, a patient with elevated blood pressure can, by a restoration of his self-esteem and by changing his attitudes toward his environment, gradually bring down the level of the blood pressure during the course of a year and a half until he functions at a level of blood pressure which can be considered appropriate.

And now, coming to the end of our story, here are a few scattered examples of other ways of reacting to stress that give rise to symptoms. I will describe an instance having to do with backache. An individual's amount of muscle tension is indicated by the firmness on palpation of the muscle. It can be shown also by a record of the actual electrical disturbance in the muscle indicating its activities. When a subject was exposed to a discussion aimed to bring into focus his feelings of hostility and anxiety, there occurred an increase in contraction of the big muscles, which were presumably contracting in readiness for action, for fight or flight. Being contracted but not actually associated with movement, they began to hurt so that the individual had backache. When he was again diverted, the activity ceased; but with a reconsideration of these threatening matters, the action potential of the muscle was again increased and again he had back pain.

Similar contraction occurs in muscles of the head. Headaches can go on for days, weeks or months, due to the sustained contraction of the sheet of muscle at the top of the head and neck when an individual is exposed to an environment which calls forth feelings of needing to be on the alert, needing to be ready to move and jump, needing to protect oneself against assaults that never quite come but always threaten. Action potential of these muscles in an individual were recorded during such a headache. A few weeks later, after he had had an opportunity to express something of his anxieties and fears and had adopted an-

other attitude, the sheet of muscle was no longer contracted, and the headache ended.

Blood vessel headaches constitute a most important aspect of man's discomfort. A person with a migraine headache may exhibit large swollen blood vessels on the side
of his head. In the same person twenty minutes later, when
the headache has been terminated, the blood vessels may
be hardly visible. You see the pertinence of this. An individual having many headaches of high intensity came to
the doctor on the first of September, told the doctor she
had bad relations with her child, and was afraid she might
murder the child. Actually, she was ashamed and fearful
of her feelings toward the child. She had no headache for
nine days after telling this story. The matter was redis-
cussed with her on the tenth day and her feelings of guilt
and hostility again were roused. A headache was precipitated. The headache was ended by the introduction of an
agent which causes swollen blood vessels to come back to
their original shape.

In another example, a similar headache was induced by
an interview with a woman about her husband, concerning whom hostile feelings were barely suppressed. During
discussion of these feelings, a headache developed as the
big arteries of her head began to throb. The pulsations of
these arteries were recorded and showed an increase in
amplitude. Now instead of using an agent causing the
blood vessels to constrict, this woman's faith in the doctor,
faith in life, faith in this representative of a constructive
life, were introduced. Then, when an intravenous injection of neutral salt-water solution was given this woman
with her new and positive attitude toward life, her headache stopped. In other words, normal salt, having no action

whatever, was capable of terminating this woman's head-ache just as a very active, constrictor agent did before.

### STOCK FACTOR AND ORGAN INFERIORITY

Why don't we all have the same bodily reactions during stress? Why do some of us get high blood pressure, others peptic ulcer, still others get ulcerative colitis, others asthma, others headache, etc.? We might as well ask, "Why are we different? Why do we look at the same assault or threat differently?" In looking at it differently, we are prepared to meet it differently. And these reactions represent our individual ways of meeting it. Do we run toward it? Do we run away from it? Do we try to avoid it? Do we try to act as though it hadn't existed? Do we wish to fight but dare not? All and more are possible ways of dealing with a threat. Now why is it that many individuals of some families have headache? Or have hypertension? Or have stomach trouble? Again, we might as well ask, "Why do dogs of certain breeds easily learn to retrieve birds? Or fight fiercely? Or follow scents? Or why do individuals of the beaver family work at building dams?"

The implication is that there are proclivities; that there are patterns which are handed down; that it's easier for a bird dog to learn to be a bird dog; that it's easier for a bulldog to hang on than it is for a cocker. Of course, it doesn't follow that the proclivity leads to disease. It only means that it's easier for an individual to meet his problems in some ways rather than in others.

A way of dealing with life is shown every day, all day, by parents, and the child gradually takes it on as his way, in addition to which he has inherited a proclivity which makes it easier for him to use a particular pattern. Thus, the individual whose parents have headache would be likely to have headache when the going is tough. But it doesn't mean that his life needs to be given over to headaches if he understands his nature, his way of looking at things, and how much of the latter has been learned from his parents.

Moreover, the repeated or prolonged participation of a given organ in a protective pattern cannot be construed as evidence of the weakness or inferiority of that organ even though, because of such participation, it fails to maintain its structural integrity. The individual may be said to be in a weak or vulnerable state, but the organ can hardly be said to be weak and, indeed, may be especially well developed and strong before it finally fails.

### CULTURE AND STRESS

Are we experiencing more stress now than ever before? Are there more stress disorders now than before? Has man never been exposed to such stress as now? That's extremely doubtful. Man has always been under stress. What then is new? What, then, creates stress for man today? A most conspicuous feature of our time is rapidity of change in customs and mores. Some cultures with opposite emphases about parents, about property, about relations of children, exhibit the same kinds of troubles that we have. Thus, it can't be just the cultural values. But any culture that's moving rapidly is one in which man's faith in his customs and habits and intuitions, his leaders and teachers and parents, is shaken. With the present cultural emphasis upon a "changing world," a man is mistakenly led to believe that the long-term values, the long-term human relationships are also changing. And therefore he loses his reference points. Furthermore, in the Western World, a man is encouraged to believe that by taking action he can find a way out of his trouble, and that by redoubling his efforts (having lost his aim), he's more likely to find a way out. The harder he tries, the more of a person he feels himself to be. And so, with this Promethean pattern, and with no guidance and with no trust, he strives, running harder—faster—without focus, without goal, without end.

Is there no light in this dark picture? No hope? Must we, then, cry out with Teiresias, about to tell Oedipus that he was doomed, "How dreadful knowledge of the truth can be when there is no help in truth"? There is help in truth. Two persons out of three exhibiting these stress manifestations can be much relieved. A responsible person of authority, who helps the sufferer regain his self-esteem, who helps him change his attitudes, can help him restore his body to more appropriate patterns of functioning.

Certainly we get courage from our knowledge that when we pursue a goal, we pay a price for it. If we know what the price is, we may then decide whether a particular goal is worth the cost. There are aims more important than comfort, and occasionally even more important than health. But an individual should know what price he is paying for his aspiration. Then, if he chooses, he may, with pain, pay for it. But he may not have all of his pie and eat it too. Often he will decide that his values are poor, or that he is confused, and change his attitudes and restore himself.

Undoubtedly, superficial mores are changing rapidly and bewilder those who cannot separate the wheat from the chaff. Such are attitudes toward property, women's place politically and economically, symbols of power and prestige, and whether one should, and to what extent, outrun his neighbor. Yet there are basic elements in human culture that fluctuate but little.

Basic cultural features concern belief in man and his constructive potential, concepts concerning men's relation to women and their respective concessions and allowances, an acceptance of parental responsibility and the giving of affection and support during the long period of childhood dependence and need for guidance, man's relation to creative effort and work, and finally, man's concept of his relation to the universe and his acceptance of his place and its pressures.

Margaret Mead suggests that in a rapidly changing culture it may be necessary for the teachers and elders to develop ways of building into individuals higher toleration for frightening circumstances than would be necessary in a more static society in which the methods for allaying fear are always present.

Could one not also hope for further help from the students of societies in giving us exact information about those aspects of human relations which change relatively little, and those that are remarkable because of their speed of rise and fall? Also, could they not indicate to us which anxiety-resolving features have the longest life and are the toughest and most capable of affording to man greater immunity to the assaults he must bear?

Much knowledge of such a nature is already in the memory and annals of man, but couched in poetic language and obsolete symbols so as to be less readily available. Perhaps with our Promethean spirit we may weld these accumulations with new knowledge and give ourselves wisdom in a culture which will probably be rapidly changing for an indefinite period of the future.

It is with this I would leave you: in times of stress we call forth bodily changes and feeling states representing a reaction to something that threatens us. What is its meaning?

What do we do about it? Do we run? Do we try to get rid of it by vomiting? Do we grimly hold on? Do we try to act as though it never was? Do we try to deal with it by non-participation? All of these reactions are associated with bodily changes of the sort I have represented and by concurrent feelings of the type which I have described. These reaction patterns evoked by stress bring a certain degree of tranquillity with them. But if used too long and obviously without solving the problem, they damage the tissue that they were aimed to preserve, and threaten the life that they were meant to prolong.

EPITOME

The stresses to which man is exposed include assaults by many living forms that aim to invade as parasites or to destroy; by meteorologic and climatic crises; by mechanical, electrical and thermal forces that operate upon man merely in terms of his mass and volume, and by elements of the earth's crust that man manipulates for his comfort and delight, or to satisfy a passion for destruction.

But constituted as he is, man is further vulnerable because he reacts not only to the actual existence of danger, but to threats and symbols of danger experienced in his past which call forth reactions little different from those to the assault itself. Since his adaptive and protective capabilities are limited, the response to many sorts of noxious agents and threats in any given man may be similar; the form of the reaction to any one agent depends more on the individual's nature and past experience than upon the particular noxious agent evoking it. Finally, because of its magnitude and duration, the adaptive-protective reaction may be far more damaging to the individual than the effects of the noxious agent per se.

Also, most important, man is a tribal or group creature with a long period of dependence and development. He is dependent for his very existence upon the aid, support and encouragement of other men. He lives his life so much in contact with men and in such concern about their expectations of him that he is jeopardized as well as supported by his fellows; indeed, he may feel more threatened by cultural and individual human pressures than by other environmental forces. He must be part of the tribe, and yet he is driven to fulfill his own proclivities. These pressures and the conflicts they engender are ubiquitous and they create a large portion of man's stress.

# "MIRACLES" — MASS PRODUCED

## By John E. McKeen

AS GREAT as the achievement has been in the field of antibiotics to date, if we step back from the swiftly moving world of our time and view this amazing progress in the perspective of the centuries, we realize that in both the scientific discovery and clinical application of antibiotics we have paced off but the first few turns of a very long road.

True, twenty-five hundred years ago, the Chinese were treating boils with the topical application of the moldy curd of the soybean. True also, a full lifetime has gone by since Pasteur learned that the common bacteria from the air could be marshalled to destroy the anthrax bacillus. Way back in 1877 he wrote prophetically that "these facts justify the highest hopes for therapeutics." In 1889 another French scientist coined the word "antibiosis," the process by which one living organism secretes a chemical discouraging to the welfare of another living organism. It was only in 1941 that Professor Selman Waksman introduced the noun "antibiotic" which is now used quite universally to refer to these microbiological antiseptic chemicals.

After Pasteur, through the years and through the decades, progress was slow and wholly exploratory. Working rationale was still lacking, the application in medicine narrowly confined. Then, very suddenly, hardly more than a decade ago, we were on the right road—our direction clearly marked.

Since 1939, we have been climbing steeply upward and at each turn, as a new vista is spread before us, confidence grows that we are on our way toward new and wondrous heights in the science of healing.

The first real glimpse of the road ahead was given to us more than twenty years ago by an eminent English research scientist. Most of you are familiar with the story of Dr. Alexander Fleming's now famous discovery, the story of a strange mold that floated in on the breeze through his laboratory window and settled on a culture of bacteria in an open petri dish. Remember, at that time, Dr. Fleming was not even looking for antibiotics. He was carrying out routine bacteriological studies. It was only through his keen observational power, combined with a fantastic chain of unlikely circumstances whereby his alert eye was drawn to the clear ring in that culture which formed about the fragment of the stray mold. It was there he caught a glimpse of that new road to antibiotic therapy. Accident? Genius? Act of God? Call it what you will, but at last we were on the way to new miracles.

After a lapse of eleven years, Dr. Howard W. Florey and his brilliant Oxford colleagues began their long, agonizing struggle to coax and to prod Fleming's mold into producing enough penicillin for clinical tests. After months of effort and tedious research, something less than a level teaspoonful of quite impure penicillin was available.

And it was just ten years ago, almost to this very day, February 12, 1941, that penicillin was administered to the first patient, an English "bobby" who had nicked himself while shaving. His head had become covered with abscesses and his entire blood stream was poisoned. Then, drop by drop, a saline solution carried penicillin into his veins. Slowly the patient emerged from a moribund condition, and for five days continued to improve. Then the supply of penicillin gave out. In an attempt to stretch their supply of this precious new drug, the ingenious Oxford scientists salvaged penicillin from the urine of the stricken man. But in spite of their unusual efforts, there was not enough penicillin. Nowhere in the world was more to be had. The infection flared again and the man died.

 In a second case, failure again resulted because supplies were inadequate. And after months of hard work, sufficient penicillin was finally accumulated to treat one more patient, a fifteen-year-old boy with a streptococcus infection that had gone far beyond the power of any other drug to combat. This boy was saved.

The accomplishments of the research scientist, Fleming, and of the research clinician, Florey, and his collaborators at Oxford, had finally bridged the gap to antibiotic therapy. But exciting as were the promises of miraculous cures, the steep road ahead threatened to keep the realization of these promises from all mankind. It appeared as though the realization of Pasteur's vision was to be reserved for still future generations.

Meanwhile the Second World War had already swept Europe. Florey saw in his mind's eye the horrible deaths resulting from the battle-wound infections—infections which accounted for half the deaths in our Civil War, and 6 per cent in World War I. He might change the course of history if only he could force a tiny organism to do his will.

Britain, writhing under the rain of Blitzkrieg fire was

fighting for its very existence. Its hospitals were crowded with war casualties. Infection was taking its toll of life and limb. Gas gangrene, abscesses, pneumonia, all these infections were probably susceptible to control by penicillin. But Britain was in no position to allocate its meagre resources to such a speculative venture, even in human therapy.

Florey, driven by his vision of miracles and accompanied by his co-worker, Norman Heatley, sought out the industrial know-how of the United States. If that great scientific discovery were to benefit humanity, it would be necessary to enlist the leaders of the American chemical industry in the adaptation of this tiny organism, *Penicillium notatum,* to the mass production methods of America. If that arsenal of democracy could turn out weapons of destruction, why could it not divert a part of its genius to the production of weapons for humanity?

When Florey reached these shores, he found that a sector of the American industry manufacturing medicinal chemicals had already caught a glimpse of his discovery. Inspired by his preliminary scientific published reports, we in America were already investigating the problem of penicillin production. He found that the American group was eager —just as eager as himself—to mitigate the evils of war with lifesaving drugs.

Three companies—Merck, Squibb, and Pfizer—and later seventeen other American manufacturers, joined with the United States Government and the English scientists in conferences to plan the production of penicillin. By the spring of 1943, America was ready to swing into full-scale production. Racing against time, manufacture began to increase sharply. In all of the previous years, the total output of penicillin had amounted to only four hundred million units, just enough for four hundred patients. By the end of the war, the yearly production rate was over seven thousand billion units—billion units, mind you—enough for over seven million patients. And then, last year American industry recorded an astounding production level of two hundred thousand billion units of penicillin. This production is approximately equal to two hundred and fifty tons of penicillin—many, many carloads for uncounted millions of patients.

Truly, in this decade of antibiotics, the achievement of the medical profession, assisted by the chemical industry, surpasses the dreams of the great Pasteur, and even those of Fleming and Florey.

But what was this production problem I have emphasized? Why was it so difficult? What were its peculiar characteristics? Let us examine them now.

In the first place, production of antibiotics led us into a new field of biochemical engineering and presented a number of entirely new problems. The basic problem was to coax this small green mold to produce penicillin under commercially practical conditions. The first penicillin produced by Florey occurred in a fermentation broth in a concentration of only about one part in a million parts of broth. Actually, there is more gold in sea water. The problem here was to extract and concentrate this valuable trace material, and to accumulate enough of it for experimental therapy. The extraction of gold from sea water would have been much simpler, because gold is fundamentally a stable element, while penicillin is one of the most fragile chemical substances ever handled by chemists. In a sentence, the task of extracting penicillin from broth was the expansion of a very sensitive microchemical laboratory procedure to an immensely larger scale production process. But now let's

look at the problem of training the living organism to produce penicillin.

The mold was grown on a solution of sugar, salt and
various other chemical nutrients. Paradoxically enough,
the major problem facing the early producers of penicillin
was to prevent the contamination of this solution by for-
eign destructive organisms. Our mold was to produce an
antibiotic which we would later use to combat these same
types of bacteria in the human system. And yet, before the
mold had a chance to grow and commence its production
of penicillin, contaminating bacteria persisted in invading
the solution to flourish there, producing substances called
penicillinase which are capable of destroying penicillin as
fast as it was being formed. Thus, the eternal warfare in the
little world of microorganisms was taking place right in
our very laboratory as we were trying to produce weapons
to combat infection. The first thing learned was that the
mold had to be grown under conditions which excluded all
other microorganisms. Conditions of sterility are comparatively easy to maintain in laboratory glassware, but in
order to get sufficient penicillin for research purposes, it
was necessary to move on a much larger scale.

Can you imagine processing fifteen hundred gallons of
broth for every person sick with infection, and doing this
under conditions which would exclude contaminating organisms which are commonly found in the air?

Penicillin was first grown in flasks, very much like milk
bottles. In fact, the first so-called bottle plant resembled
milk-bottling plants to a great degree. It was soon realized,
however, that if we were to procure the desired amount of
penicillin, we would have to erect bottle plants greater in
capacity than all of the milk-bottling plants in the United
States combined, and would have to process six million

*John E. McKeen*

flasks every month, obviously impossible. Therefore, fermentation chemists turned to cultivation of the penicillin mold in a submerged aerated condition in large tanks.

In the early deep tank production, penicillin for one patient required the aeration of broth with approximately ten times the air contained in this auditorium. Moreover, air for antibiotic production must be completely sterilized. When one considers a recent scientific report that with each breath of air we breathe in New York City, we draw in 185,000 particles of dust, the enormity of sterilizing thousands of cubic feet of air per minute for our fermentations can be thoroughly realized.

But the problem of penicillin fermentation was not simply the mechanical multiplication of laboratory conditions to large scale. Just as the farmer fertilizes crops for greater productivity, so the fermentation chemist added mold nutrients to give higher yields of penicillin. This fertilization of the mold was made even more effective as the organic chemist determined the molecular structure of penicillin. Based on this structural knowledge, the fermentation chemist was then able to add small fragments of the penicillin molecule readily prepared by man to aid the mold in its antibiotic production.

Other teams of Government and industry scientists were searching for new strains of the penicillin mold which might produce larger quantities than Fleming's original mold. They looked everywhere, and strangely enough, one day as they walked through the streets of Peoria, one of the Government scientists picked up a moldy canteloupe—the kind that one would throw away—and when this mold was taken into the laboratory, it was found to increase production of penicillin as much as fivefold.

All of these scientific accomplishments I have enumer-

138

ated enabled the American chemical industry to deliver the necessary quantity of penicillin to the beachhead in Normandy on D-Day.

Continuing their research after the war, the organic chemists finally crystallized penicillin in an exceptionally pure form. Today, this is the product your doctor prescribes for you.

This penicillin story has shown the indispensable role of the research scientist whose discovery made possible the accomplishments of chemotherapy; of the research clinician whose courageous and patient studies have demonstrated the value of penicillin; and finally of the American chemical industry which solved the problem of production and brought penicillin in quantity to the soldier and civilian alike. We are humbly proud of our accomplishment of multiplying the original teaspoonful of penicillin to the tons of pure crystalline drug now available to everyone on prescription not only in America but in every country throughout the free world.

But penicillin is only one brilliant chapter in the story of the decade of antibiotics. You know that in recent years a number of other antibiotics have been discovered and developed to increase the physician's armamentarium in his battle against infection. In 1944, Professor Waksman announced the discovery of streptomycin. In a few short years, the medical investigators had established its usefulness in the chemotherapy of tuberculosis. It was the first substance promising any value in the treatment of this scourge. Today one hundred tons of streptomycin per year are being used by the medical profession all over the world, in the treatment of tuberculosis and other diseases not affected by penicillin.

The next chapter in the decade of antibiotics, and one

that gives even greater hope for the future, has been marked by the development of antibiotics with a broader range of effectiveness. As wonderful as penicillin was, there were a number of bacterial infections it could not control. Because its range of effectiveness is confined to a specific class of bacteria, it is termed a narrow-spectrum antibiotic.

Streptomycin also had a narrow spectrum which fortunately did not overlap, but extended beyond, the range of penicillin. However, even the combined range of penicillin and streptomycin left many infections still to be conquered. Most of the infections controlled by penicillin and streptomycin are bacterial in nature. Beyond this group, however, are many infections caused by even smaller microorganisms, called the rickettsiae and viruses.

The narrow-spectrum antibiotics were totally ineffective against this group of small organisms. But the research scientist pushed on again. Spurred by the initial successes and learning slowly but well the lessons of the first two antibiotics, the team of the research scientists, medical clinicians, and industrial technologists, rapidly extended control to other human infections.

In 1947, Burkholder announced the discovery of chloramphenicol. In 1948, Duggar discovered aureomycin; in 1950, a team of research scientists of Chas. Pfizer & Co., of which I am a part, announced the discovery of the newest broad-spectrum antibiotic, terramycin.

These three antibiotics, chloramphenicol, aureomycin and terramycin are termed broad-spectrum antibiotics because they not only control the range of infection previously treated by penicillin and streptomycin but they have also extended the range of control into infections caused by rickettsiae and certain viruses. The extent of this broader range is appreciated when it is realized that penicillin is

useful in the treatment of approximately twenty-five different infections; streptomycin is useful in the treatment of
fifteen infections; but terramycin and the other broad-
spectrum antibiotics are useful in the treatment of more
than fifty infections.

You will remember that some fifteen years elapsed between the first scientific recognition of penicillin as an antibiotic and the achievements of the large-scale production of
this drug. In view of this, it is remarkable that in the last
three years of the decade of antibiotics a new antibiotic has
been discovered and has reached large-scale production and
widespread clinical usefulness in each of these last three
years. The entire development of terramycin from the time
it was isolated from the soil to the final large-scale production, and including a thoroughgoing clinical testing period,
required less than one year.

I call to your attention this contrast with penicillin, not
merely as a striking illustration of the use of accumulated
foreknowledge, but because I think this accomplishment
has an important bearing on the chemical industry's future
contributions to human welfare. There is no reason to
assume that the exploratory range in chemotherapy, even
on the level of basic principles, has now been exhausted.
Only minds which have become susceptible to the comforts
of entrenchment seem to dwell on that illusion. It is quite
possible that one day a discovery as sweeping as antibiosis
may yet be announced; but in such an event, the working
team drawn from scientific research, industrial technology
and clinical practice, will be better prepared to solve the
problems of application than were those lone workers who
have beaten their separate paths through the maze of other
years.

As in chemicals, so in the working of men's minds, there

### John E. McKeen

is a synergistic pyramiding wherein they combine to great effect, achieving beyond the sum of their separate capacities. Most often the difference lies in the time it takes to attain the aspirations of mankind, but in medicine, this is measurable not only in years, but by the fateful yardstick of needless suffering and even of untimely death. We cannot say, of course, that from here on out we shall always be able to telescope the difficult task into such a short period. But what we do say is that through the interplay of specialized ability, we have removed many of the road blocks of the past. It is in the broad fields of research and production that the teaming up of these abilities is so important to the clinical enterprise pioneering in new ground.

The discovery and development of terramycin has been an outstanding example of the teamwork of many branches of science. Without the synergism of all the scientific minds involved, it might have taken years to bring forth terramycin instead of the months that elapsed from its discovery to clinical usefulness.

The teamwork began in the search for new antibiotic-producing molds. In this culture screening program, we no longer had to depend on the chance discovery of a moldy canteloupe, or the agency of a stray breeze. We actually made a systematic search of the soil, which is the most fruitful source of organisms producing antibiotics. From all over the world to our biochemical research laboratories came samples of earth. Thousands each month from travelers, missionaries and overseas air line pilots. These soil samples were suspended in water, and the liquid poured on petri dishes, then allowed to incubate at a warm temperature. After a few days, colonies grew on those plates and random samples were selected and placed in test tubes for further study.

A screening test was then run on each selected colony. Here again the petri dish was employed and the selected mold was grown in the presence of numerous pathogenic organisms. In this work, the mycologists observed many hundreds of times daily the clear ring around the molds that first gave Fleming his clue to penicillin.

This is how the mycologists, those experts on molds, began the search for terramycin. These procedures are being repeated many times over every day in industrial laboratories throughout the country.

It might sound peculiar to you, but one of the hardest jobs of this antibiotic search was to identify quickly the already known antibiotics and eliminate them from consideration. In this work a new technique, known as paper chromatography, proved exceedingly useful.

As soon as the antimicrobial activity of the selected mold was established and it was felt that it might represent a new antibiotic, the next member of the team, the biochemist, then took over. He studied the fermentation characteristics of the mold, and prepared small samples of antibiotics for further testing. His research work on the new antibiotic represents the area where nearly all of the hurdles must be cleared and, conversely, where most of the candidates for further testing are completely eliminated.

In animals such as rabbits and mice, acute toxicity, chronic toxicity, damage to the nervous system, kidney damage, liver damage and allergic reactions were examined. All of these represent road blocks which had to be successfully cleared by the new antibiotic.

At this point, it was important to begin the development of the biological assay for the new antibiotic. It originally occurred in such an impure form that a simple chemical test was not possible; therefore, it was necessary, on the

*143*

basis of the antimicrobial characteristics of the drug, to select a bacterial strain which could be used to measure the activity of the sought-for antibiotic under a wide variety of conditions. Until such a biological assay was evolved, very little future progress could be made in the evaluation of the antibiotic.

As soon as this hurdle had been cleared, the medical bacteriologists stepped in and set up animal protection studies. The object of these studies was to see if infections in animals could be prevented or cured by the new drug. After the medical bacteriologist issued an encouraging report, the fermentation and organic chemists studied the development of large-scale production of the yet unnamed antibiotic.

It was one thing to search the fifty-six million square miles of the earth's land area for that certain handful of soil; it was still another to pick certain microorganisms out of that particular handful; and it was yet another to put that organism to work in a large-scale plant.

It was now the objective of the chemical team to produce the antibiotic in pure crystalline form, since it is only under those conditions that the most favorable performance could be achieved. Terramycin was finally isolated in pure canary yellow crystals.

Still another member of the team stepped in at this point, the pharmaceutical chemist. In order to increase the antimicrobial performance of antibiotics, it is necessary to maintain a pharmaceutical laboratory for the preparation of numerous dosage forms, such as capsules, tablets, ointments, elixir, troches, ophthalmic, intravenous, and dental preparations. Because of terramycin's excellent chemical stability, it lent itself to all these dosage forms.

At this point, the last but most important member of the

research team took over, the medical clinician. It was then necessary to determine in human patients the validity of the animal tests. Modern clinicians demand that any new drug meet very rigid pharmacological specifications and insist on very thorough animal tests to assure safety of administration to human patients.

When the clinician was satisfied that no possibility of damage to the patient exists, clinical trials were agreed upon. These were guided by the animal work of the medical bacteriologists. All but a few of terramycin's laboratory indications against diseases were definitely established by the clinicians in human therapy.

Terramycin was found to have a decisive inhibitory effect on staphylococci in cases of septicemia, meningitis, osteomyelitis, abscesses, and other infections; and on streptococci in cases of meningitis, tonsillitis, septic sore throat, scarlet fever, erysipelas, and bacterial endocarditis, a severe infection of the heart. Also in the clinically verified spectrum were virus pneumonia, gonorrhea and syphilis, bacillary and amoebic dysentery, tularemia, anthrax, gas gangrene, typhus, scrub typhus, Rocky Mountain spotted fever and rickettsial pox; and the drug worked miracles in clearing up the ravages of the human body caused by the tropical infection of yaws.

With an antibiotic of such great promise, it was necessary to proceed very quickly to large-scale production in order to supply the tremendous demands of the medical profession for such a useful drug.

In contrast to the early deep tanks of penicillin production, terramycin is now produced in tremendous fermentation vats that would reach from the floor to the ceiling of this auditorium. The air requirements of the terramycin production fermentation plant are so great that our air

*John E. McKeen*

compressor installation rivals those of a large steel blast furnace. Before the antibiotic can be extracted, the wrinkled mold, streptomyces rimosus, which produces terramycin, must be removed from the broth. This is accomplished on huge rotary filters which are engineering devices for the separation of solids from liquids. Then begins the long, tedious process of extraction and purification of terramycin.

When the canary yellow crystals have been obtained, various dosage forms of terramycin are prepared. Some of these forms require handling under sterile conditions to prevent the slightest contamination. These dosage forms are then packaged and prepared for distribution.

Even at this point, scientific teamwork does not end. Before any antibiotic can leave our plant, it is necessary for it to pass rigid quality control specifications to insure its safety and efficacy when used on human patients.

This complex production process must be carefully integrated and controlled to assure efficient mass production. It is typical of the antibiotic industry, through large expenditures for research and process development, to decrease progressively the cost of antibiotics through mass production. This has already been accomplished in the case of penicillin and streptomycin. Substantial improvements in antibiotic processing will give reasonable assurance of declining prices for the newer antibiotics, even in the face of current inflationary trends.

However, terramycin is but a chapter in the great antibiotic story. More important than the discovery of terramycin, and the uses of penicillin and all the other known antibiotics, is the great potential area of chemotherapy which remains up to now unknown.

Antibiotics have enabled our doctors to cut nearly in half the death rate from pneumonia. They can safeguard

*146*

humanity from the once terrifying effects of many conta-
gions; they can save millions of lives through the recovery
from wounds without handicap of infection. They can, in
time, practically eliminate the scourge of venereal diseases.

But there is much more that antibiotics might do. The
incentive to expand these researches is tremendous, for
among the diseases which are still beyond the control of
any known antibiotic are several of high incidence, such as
the common cold, measles, chickenpox, mumps, and malaria, and several others of grave consequence—cancer and
poliomyelitis.

The great challenge to antibiotic therapy that still remains is epitomized by another scientific accomplishment
of the past decade. Florey was driven to further research by
his mental picture of the terrible toll of infection occa-
sioned by war wounds. Likewise, it is now ominous, but
true, that research to control postirradiation infection from
atomic blasts ought to be pursued with the same drive, the
same teamwork, the same dedicated spirit that turned penicillin into a clinical reality.

Antibiotics give promise of developing successful therapy
and even effective prophylaxis for protection against the
aftermath of atomic warfare. The promise of alleviation
from the terrible effects of this dreaded weapon places an
additional responsibility on the shoulders of the antibiotic
industry. And I want to assure you that even now we are
providing for vastly increased terramycin facilities. By the
end of this year we shall have doubled our capacity to produce this new wonder drug. This expansion, combined
with strategic dispersal of antibiotic production facilities
into three widely separated plants, should assure adequate
supplies in the event of a national emergency—an emergency we fervently hope will never occur.

*John E. McKeen*

In fields other than therapeutics, antibiotics evidence additional usefulness. It has been discovered that when continuously fed at low level, antibiotics increase the growth of poultry, swine and calves. This effect increases our available food supply and makes the utilization of more abundant animal feedstuffs possible—important factors as we face increasing food demands and rising prices.

Thus, as we celebrate the first decade of antibiotics, we look back upon accomplishments unprecedented in medical history. A noteworthy degree of scientific teamwork in research, in production, and in clinical application has already been achieved. The research scientist has given us new discoveries; the production engineer has given us mass production know-how; and the clinician has utilized these mass-produced miracle drugs for the alleviation of human suffering throughout the world.

In the forthcoming decade of antibiotics, no doubt, new and significant discoveries will be made. Indeed, in the industry's laboratories, we are finding hints of things to come—discoveries which may help to deal with serious diseases which yet remain unconquered. Production will not lag behind research; and as fast as these new discoveries come, we shall do our utmost to make them available through the physician to all of the people. Each of us can look forward to longer and, I trust, better lives because of antibiotics—miracles, mass produced.

*Index*

# INDEX

ACTH, 36-38
  "era of," 32-33
  *see also* Hormones
Adaptation
  chain reaction of, 36
"Adapation syndrome," 32-33, 51
  *see also* "General adaptation
    syndrome"
Adaptability
  as a great force, 34-35
Aggression
  in animals, 70-71
  and domination, 67-71
  and sex, 71
Airways
  in relation to stress and emo-
    tions, 114-120
Alarm reactions, 34
Allee, W. C., 73
Animal psychology, 8
  attitude toward, 44
  in relation to psychiatry, 45-72
Animals
  experiments on, 34, 45, 47
  in antibiotic research, 143-145
  negativism in, 72
  neurosis in, 46, 61-63
  psychology of, 8
  psychosis of, 63
  primary needs of, 64-68
  *see also* Chimpanzees, Dogs,
    Monkeys, Pigs, and Rats
Antiaircraft defense, 14-15, 22
Antibiotics
  and chemotherapy, 86-88
  development of therapy of, 8
  discovery of, 80, 133
  future of, 90-92, 147-148
  kinds of, 88-90

mass production of, 9
producing molds for, 142-143
quest for, 8, 76-92
significance of terms for, 78
what they are, 77
where found, 78
*see also* ACTH, Aureomycin,
  Chloramphenicol, Cortisone,
  DAC, GC., Penicillin, MC,
  Streptomycin, STH, Terramycin
Arthritic and rheumatic disorders, 37
Asthma, 118
Attitudes
  in relation to stress, emotions
    and bodily disease, 106-107
  toward animal psychology, 44
Aureomycin, 140, 141
Automatic control system, 20, 23
  *see also* Machines

Babies, *see* Children
Backache, 124
Baron, A. L., 93
Bayne-Jones, S., 4
Beach, F. A., 73
Bernard, C., 7, 20, 39
Bickford, 21
Bigelow, J., 15
Bird, C., 73
Birds
  organic needs of, 64
  experiments with, 61-62
  *see also* Chickens
Blood pressure, *see* Heart
Bodily changes
  interpretation of, 112

# Index

Engines
steering, 16
*see also* Machines
Environment
fitness of, 19
Exhaustion, 34
Experimental neurosis, *see* Neurosis
Experimental studies
compared to clinical, 53-56
Experimentation
versus natural observation, 45

Feedback, 16-19
Fire control, 15
Fleming, A., 79, 82, 134, 136, 138, 143
discovers antibiotics, 132
Florey, H. W., 82, 93, 133-136
Freud, S., 39, 48
Frustration
experiments in, 58

Gadget
and human beings, 25
Galdston, I., 4
G-C., 38
*see also* Antibiotics
Gantt, W. H., 73
"General adaptation syndrome," 33-34, 42
*see also* "Adaptation Syndrome"
Gilbraiths
system of, 24
Gosio, 81
Grace, W. J., 100, 106, 120
Graham, D., 95, 100, 106
Groen, J., 120

Hay fever, 115
Headaches, 124-125, 127
Heart, 122-124
Heatley, N., 135
Hens, *see* Chickens
Hench, P. S., 37, 43
Henderson, 19
Herrick, H. T., 93
Hetrick, J. A. W., 4
Hippocrates, 31
Hoarding, 55
Holmes, 120
Homeostasis, 7
Homeostat, 20-22
Hoppe-Seyler, E. F., 81
Hormones
"adaptive," 33
corticotrophic, 36, 42
*see also* ACTH
Hotchkiss, R. D., 82
Human relations
in relation to stress, 127-131
Hunt, J. McV., 53, 73

Industrial revolution, 24
Irving, G. W., 93

Katz, D., 74
Kellogg and Kellogg, 74
Kendall, E. S., 43
Keyes, H. B., 4
Klee, J. B., 74
Knowledge
and wisdom, 31-32
Köhler, W., 74
Kruse, H. D., 4

Laity Lectures
aim of, 7
Leisure, 27
Levy, D. M., 8, 44-75
Liddell, H. S., 59, 74
Life situations
in relation to emotions and bodily disease, 8

# Index

Machines
    computing, 13
    homeostatic, 22
    limitations of, 35
    moral problem of, 27
    of control and communication,
        25
    *see also* Engines, Feedback,
        Homeostats
Maier, N. R. F., 74
Marie, P., 42
Maslow, A. H., 74
Massachusetts Institute of Tech-
    nology, 7
Masserman, J. H., 74
Maternal drive, 68
Maxwell, C., 16
Mayo Clinic, 21
M-C, 38
McKeen, J. E., 8, 9, 132-148
Mead, M., 129
Medical research, 35, 40-41
Medicine
    types of advances in, 31
"Men, Machines, and the World
    About," 7, 13-29
Merck, and Co., 135
Method and theory
    limitations of, 47-48
Microorganisms, 78, 91
Middle Ages, 28
Mineralo-corticoids, *see* Corti-
    coids
Mobilization patterns
    in relation to stress and emo-
        tions, 122
Monkeys, 62-63, 65, 69-71
Moss, F. A., 74
Mowrer, O. H., 74

Nasal membrane, *see* Airways

Nature
    "bookkeeping" and "landscap-
        ing" of, 32
Negativism, 72-73
Neurosis
    experimental, 58-61
New York Academy of Medicine,
    4, 7, 30
Noxious stimuli
    in inducing stress, 34
Noble, R. C., 74

Objectivity, 40
Observation
    natural, versus experimental,
        45
Organ inferiority, 126-127

Pasteur, L., 39, 81, 132, 134, 136
Pavlov, I. P., 39, 47, 58-60, 75
Pavlovianism, 8
Peightal, T. C., 4
Penicillin
    discovery of, 79, 133
    first administered, 133-135
    increased production of, 36-39
    uses of, 140-141
    *see also* Antibiotics
Peptides, 82
Pfizer, Chas. & Co., 8, 135, 140
Pig, 46
Polly, H. F., 43
Pratt, R., 93
Psychoanalysis, 48-53
Psychiatry
    in relation to psychology, 8, 44
Psychodynamics, 63-73
Psychology, *see* Animal psy-
    chology
Psychopathology
    and clinical neurosis, 61-63
Psychoses, 63

154